Communicating Care

THE LANGUAGE OF NURSING

Paul Crawford
Former Lecturer in Mental Health, University of Birmingham

Brian Brown
Lecturer in Psychology and Sociology, De Montfort University

Peter Nolan
Senior Lecturer in the School of Health Sciences, University of Birmingham

Stanley Thornes (Publishers) Ltd

First published 1998 by
Stanley Thornes Publishers Ltd
Ellenborough House
Wellington Street
Cheltenham
GL50 1YW
UK

610.73069 CRA

ISBN 0 7487 3306 X

98 99 00 01 02 / 10 9 8 7 6 5 4 3 2 1

SMC

Typeset by WestKey Limited, Falmouth, Cornwall
Printed and bound in Great Britain by TJ International Ltd., Padstow, Cornwall

CONTENTS

For Jamie Orion

The warrior stood
At the old ford
Black-feathered with crows
Eyes of uric
Immortal

ACKNOWLEDGEMENTS

We would like to thank Alison J. Johnson for her contribution to our arguments concerning narrative and genre in chapters 1 and 2, respectively, and to our analysis of nursing language in chapter 3. We would like to thank Karen D. Richards for her analysis of nursing student responses to case vignettes in chapter 6. Thanks are also extended to our editor, Tony Wayte, who endeavoured to bring our project to the boil and provided much encouragement and support. Finally, we are grateful to the anonymous reviewer for their most helpful and generous remarks.

PREFACE

This book aims to assist nurses in understanding the way in which the language of nursing shapes their relationships with colleagues and clients and defines the work they do. We shall demonstrate the various forms language can take and the purposes for which it is used. There is at present no other book that addresses all the issues we intend to cover in this book or that draws together the growing body of research on the language of caring. So far, a number of surveys, analyses and guidelines for practice have been published which have looked at the importance of language in nursing. The aim of this book is to consolidate and add to this work so that all nurses can understand its relevance to their own practice. Many theories of language emphasize how powerful it is; this book shows nurses how they can wield that power. It places the language debate firmly in the arena of practice, promoting not so much a model of nursing language but a raised awareness of what individual nurses can achieve by what they say and write, and by how they respond to what they hear and read.

Nurses will need little reminding of the steady progress made by their profession during the last three decades. Only a century ago, the work of nurses was closely linked to the running of institutions, be they infirmaries or asylums. For the most part, nursing work meant ensuring cleanliness, maintaining order and, above all, carrying out medical orders (Rafferty, 1996). The emphasis on routine and task-led care became so entrenched that by the early 1960s Menzies (1961) observed that nurses devoted more energy to routines than to the human needs of their patients. This situation continued until the 1970s, when communication skills, psychology and sociology were introduced into all basic training programmes for nurses. Recent research (Kitson, 1993) has confirmed the importance of the nurse's personal relationship with the patient and the patient's relatives; this relationship is seen as the cornerstone of care, contributing immensely to the overall well-being of the patient. The nursing literature now reflects nurses' commitment to the quality of interpersonal relations in their work.

Critical and analytical skills are needed if the nurse is to be able to reflect on the relationships he or she establishes with patients or clients and thereby evaluate the quality of care provided. Reflective practice is increasingly hailed as the hallmark of a mature professional who is responsibly engaged in promoting the best interests of those they care for. This book seeks to contribute to the maturing of the nursing profession by emphasizing the importance of nursing language as a tool of reflective practice. Nowadays, an awareness of the use and misuse of language is essential in order to engage in reflective practice. Language issues include consideration of such key areas as how nurses talk about their work, how they write about what they have done, and how nursing is defined by employers, managers, educationalists, lawyers and patients.

The book provides a starting point in the journey towards acquiring competency in the philosophy and theory of language. It will describe the work that has already been done on the language of doctor–patient interactions, and studies that have been carried out by social workers, occupational therapists, psychiatrists and many other carers as well as by nurses. A large amount of material generated in many different disciplines will be presented in a way that should be easily accessible to nursing students and nurse lecturers. It is important to acknowledge and explore the work that has been done on the language of health care in so many different fields because we want to emphasize how the same language processes are common to different kinds of health care interaction. A second reason for trying to increase nurses' understanding of language by referring to the care provided by other health professionals is because nursing has only recently started to develop its own theories of care, and nurses are still relative newcomers in the research arena.

Nurses are more and more accustomed to working in multidisciplinary teams and to providing many different kinds of care, from supportive psychotherapy to aiding the rehabilitation of people with head injuries. This is a far cry from the era of task-orientated care and the taking of temperatures and emptying of bedpans. Nurses need to understand how their language of care is now shared by many different carers. This book helps the reader explore the language operating in the context of many different health care tasks and make comparisons with how nurses talk to and with patients.

The aim of the book is to simplify language theory whilst retaining a sense of its richness, and thereby to make it less intimidating but not less fascinating for the reader. Many of the books and journal articles written about language are not aimed at a nursing audience, so nursing students and nurse lecturers find it difficult to relate to developments in discourse analysis, sociolinguistics, philosophy, psychology and psychiatry which are nonetheless highly applicable to their own discipline. This book will provide many different examples of nursing language in action to enable nurses to feel as confident in their understanding of language as other professionals – after all, nurses spend much more time speaking to clients and writing about them than most other groups of carers. The book aims to show nurses how effective language can be in disseminating their view of health care and in challenging inappropriate representations of the people they care for.

The book will confront the difficulties that the language of nursing often creates, especially when words lead to deeds with unacceptable consequences for those receiving care. The way in which nurses talk and write about those they care for will be described and analysed, fusing the theory and practice of nursing language so as to appeal to all nurses, whether clinicians, educators or managers.

Chapter 1 introduces the reader to language as a kind of social action. It explores nursing texts and how professional bodies have sought to regulate the style and content of these texts. The aim is to help nurses understand how human beings characteristically embed their experiences in narratives and how it is necessary to understand such narratives if we are to grasp what the patient's illness means to him or her and what nursing means to nurses. The rhetoric of 'helping' is examined in order to expose the gloss placed on caring activities which conceals the oppression of patients.

Chapter 2 examines whether the person writing is the sole author of his or her words and how what he or she writes is inevitably informed by politics, economics and the need to explain the patient's distress. The culture in which patients have grown up and in which they have learnt to experience their bodies and minds will be noted as having a crucial role to play in how they present their illnesses and in what they tell their nurses. How the patient's account is translated into patient records depends on a whole range of workplace decision-making strategies and record-keeping routines which ultimately result in records being woefully incomplete. Nurses are constantly exhorted to keep better records, but the gaps in the records will not be filled in simply by telling people to fill them. Only by understanding the reasons for incomplete record keeping can the problem be addressed with any chance of success.

Chapter 3 develops the idea that the language used in health care settings forms a distinctive genre, a unique way of talking and writing. It considers how nursing students are encouraged to put on a linguistic uniform so as to be able to address the problems patients present them with and to provide the solutions that the health care system has to offer. Communication in health care settings is influenced by a huge range of factors, from the overall political structure of health care to the type of forms on which patients' records are kept. The kind of 'linguistic entrapment' to which nurses are subject also restricts what patients can tell us about themselves, and their records may bear little relation to their own perception of their problems.

Chapter 4 deals with the thorny question of meaning. Most of us can distinguish what is meaningful from mere gibberish, yet defining meaning can be very difficult indeed. Meaning is something that groups of people create as they strive to make sense of the world. Meaning can be ascribed to bodily and mental symptoms, to encounters with colleagues and patients and to our work in health care. However, meaning is often contested, particularly when people debate what it means to be ill, nor is the meaning of illness always defined by health professionals. Patients may organize themselves to demand that their point of view be taken seriously; this is how ME and seasonal affective disorder came to be recognized and accepted. In order to generate meaning in health care, research reports, textbooks and even medical or nursing notes have to hide the author so that they look as if they simply describe the world as it is. In order to make sense of the world, personal identity and differences of opinion may have to be suppressed.

Chapter 5 looks at how the language used in health care settings is carefully selected to win over those who are intended to hear it – in other words the audience – be they patients, clients or professional colleagues. The business of making sense of language is by no means straightforward, as many interpretations are possible; in fact, the language of health care and the settings in which health care is provided limit the meanings that can be deduced. The settings in which nursing is carried out are bursting with a whole variety of speakers and writers, hearers and readers. The talk and writing of nurses depends on who they are and the people they are communicating with. Nurses do not tell doctors to do things but they might make suggestions. Managers have their own way of trying to win staff round to their point of view, just as ward sisters and doctors have a tendency to fight their corners. In some cases, such as when patients are being treated against their will, the process of health care is facilitated by people who deliberately insulate themselves from the patients' views.

Chapter 6 discusses how the complex, multi-authored biographies of patients written by health professionals may be detrimental to patients. For example: the way staff reason about patients and make sense of their conditions may be affected by racial stereotypes so that ethnic minorities are perceived to be more violent and less open to counselling than white clients. This chapter also explores the issue of 'secondary baby talk', which is sometimes used by health professionals when they are talking to elderly patients. The effect of such language in consolidating the incapacity of the elderly is considered.

Finally, chapter 7 draws together the implications for health care practitioners and students of the richly textured linguistic environment in which they work, be it a hospital, GP surgery or the community. The implications of the language we use in terms of being able to engage in reflective practice are discussed at length. If reflection is to be taken seriously, it must involve a critical awareness of the power of language, as language is the very foundation of health care. We argue that if reflective practice is to become a powerful learning tool then it is the responsibility of every nurse to assume responsibility for acquiring as much understanding of the power of language as possible.

REFERENCES

Kitson, A. (1993) *Nursing: Art and Science*, Chapman & Hall, London.
Menzies, I. (1961) The functioning of social systems as a defence against anxiety. *Human Relations*, **13**, 95–121.
Rafferty, A.M. (1996) *The Politics of Nursing Knowledge*, Routledge, London.

1 LANGUAGE ACTS: IT'S THE WAY YOU TELL THEM

AIMS

This chapter introduces some of the major issues in language relating to health care settings, in order to help the reader to gain an appreciation of the importance of language in the provision of high-quality care. This chapter will also show that language is fundamentally an activity; it is a way of doing things and getting others to do them.

We will stress that language has the power to harm as well as to heal and that responsible practitioners should be aware that patients may be devalued or undermined by the terms used to describe them.

We aim to show that critical language theory and postmodernism can inform our understanding of the varied roles language plays in health care. The language of nursing may take the form of informal stories about patients or the more formal processes of record keeping. Whereas professional bodies such as the UKCC offer guidelines about record keeping, everyday communication is less frequently addressed.

Patients and professionals use language to construct narratives of health and illness which enable them to make sense of the illness experience. But also language can lead to actions that may not be in the patient's interests, and can recast oppressive practices as therapeutic ones.

Throughout the book we will be picking out some papers and books written by other authors which we have found particularly useful or influential – our 'key references'. These will be listed separately at the end of each chapter. If the reader (or indeed the educator) has the opportunity, reading these will give a flavour of the background material on which our thinking is based.

INTRODUCTION: COMMUNICATING CARE

Nursing is fundamentally about *communicating care*. It involves doing things to and for people, but at its very heart it involves informing people about what is being done to them and why, and discussing with them the likely consequences of health care interventions. Language has always been central to the theory and practice of nursing care. Much of nursing is about communicating in day-to-day spoken and written interactions with staff, patients and relatives. This might take place in such activities as counselling, patient records or care planning. Conscientious practitioners are always reflecting on how they communicate with others and how they talk or write about the way they deliver care. Yet there has been little guidance for nurses about the language they use and how that language is central to their practice; how it can both help and hinder their work, and is situated among and sometimes in conflict with many other competing languages in the health care industry as a whole.

Although nursing language might generally be thought of as useful, practical and informative, this is not always the case. In fact, words and phrases used by nurses, as with other health professionals, can be damaging. The motto 'sticks and stones may break my bones but words will never hurt me' is plainly wrong. Inappropriate and insensitive nursing language can and does hurt. Since nursing is typically viewed as a caring profession which promotes the health and well-being of individuals, it may seem offensive to suggest that nurses are sometimes guilty of using language that is abusive or damaging. However, to ignore the potential for language to be harmful and to focus purely on the positive aspects of nursing talk and writing would be to miss an opportunity for professional development and growth. Dwight

Key reference

Bolinger (1980) claims that language can be thought of as a 'loaded weapon' beyond the rule of law: 'Loaded language, like loaded fire-arms, can be hidden where least suspected, and the laws against concealed weapons do not apply' (p. 88).

Language is not neutral, Bolinger argues, but 'a thousand ways biased' (p. 68). The power of language to dominate others has been

Key reference

further investigated by Norman Fairclough (1989). He argues for greater attention to be paid to the power of language and advocates critical language study (CLS) 'to help increase consciousness of how language contributes to the domination of some people by others, because consciousness is the first step towards emancipation' (p. 1). Fairclough considers that there is no 'critical consciousness' about the talk and writing that is specific to nurses or what can be called 'nursing's discourse'. He writes:

> Workers are currently being subjected to enormous pressure to adapt their practices in order to meet the purely instrumental criteria of bureaucratic rationality, such as 'efficiency' and 'cost-effectiveness'. And for many of them this means that fewer workers are expected to 'handle' more people. Consequently, in so far as discourse or 'communication' figure in training, they tend to figure in the form of 'communication' or 'social skills' whose primary motivation is efficient people-handling . . . CLS could be a significant resource for those who are concerned about such developments. (p. 235)

In this book we hope to go a long way to correcting the lack of 'critical consciousness' about the language of nursing. Fairclough's comments indicate quite strongly that nursing language does not work in isolation from wider political and economic directives or, indeed, fashions. As it competes with the languages of other health care professionals, such as doctors, psychologists, occupational therapists and so on, it also struggles to remain autonomous within an increasingly market-driven health care system. Here it would be as well to say something about the concept of 'ideology' itself and, indeed, competing 'ideologies', because, as we shall reveal, nursing language is bound up with powerful conceptions of how our society should be constructed and run.

IDEOLOGIES OF LANGUAGE, IDEOLOGIES OF NURSING

The concept of 'ideology' is central to the study of language and has preoccupied scholars since the nineteenth century. It underlies much of the thinking about language which will form the basis of this book. The term 'ideology' was first used at the beginning of the nineteenth century to refer to a science of ideas (Billig, 1982; Graumann, 1984). However, by the time it appeared in the work of political thinkers like Marx and Engels in the mid-nineteenth century, it referred specifically to a false body of ideas. At that time, it was considered natural that society ran along clearly defined lines which placed rich and powerful people at the top of the social order. Marx and Engels disagreed with the notion that this represented the natural state of affairs, and considered that this dominant ideology or false body of ideas was imposed on society by powerful class interests (Therborn, 1980).

In much contemporary thinking, the term 'ideology' is used to refer to the myths, images, and representations of reality which hold society together. People may make use of ideologies to help them understand their world (Jensen, 1987). Frazer (1987) offers the following definition: '[An ideology is] a coherent body or system of ideas, typically about the public realm or man's place in it, whose origin and existence are explicable by reference to the social position and interests of some group' (p. 409). There are many examples of people being greatly influenced by the ideologies with which they come into contact. For example, the lives of people in China are influenced by the ideas of Communism. In the USA the idea of the free market dominates and shapes the lives of its people. Equally, nursing is shaped by powerful ideologies such as the bureaucratic 'cost-effectiveness' and 'efficiency' that Fairclough mentions. We might also think about the ideology of self-care in the health industry. This emphasis on the individual's responsibility for their health is not neutral or non-political. It shapes the way that nurses themselves approach those in their care. The biomedical model or approach to care is another ideology. Other ideologies such as psychosocial models of care or those that promote alternative therapies are displaced by this powerful body of ideas. As another theorist, Peter Leonard (1984), puts it, 'Ideologies . . . both subject us to the social order and prepare (or qualify) us for participation in it by telling us (a) what exists and what nature, society, men and women are like, (b) what is good, right, just, beautiful and enjoyable and its opposites, and (c) what is possible and impossible' (p. 106).

The notion of ideology helps us to grasp the role of the state in the lives of individuals. Various theorists (Stedman-Jones, 1971; Dale, 1976; Wilson, 1977; Ginsburg, 1980; Parry, Rustin and Satyamurti, 1979) have noted the effects of state intervention in the form of social welfare programmes. These programmes have had a direct material impact on the recipients of welfare and a more subtle ideological effect in subjecting many families to state regulation. Nurses, social workers and the police, to name just a few groups, may all play a part in diffusing mainstream ideas and models of conduct through the various social strata with which they come into contact. The role of the state in influencing the way that we organize our lives is difficult to deny. This is relevant to nursing because nurses may be carrying out activities that are not compatible with their profession's or their own value systems. Nurses are compelled to accept large-scale changes in the way health care is delivered. For example, nurses may believe that health care should be delivered 'from the cradle to the grave', and yet state initiatives have dramatically altered this principle over recent years. Increasingly, health and social welfare are privatized, individualized and left to the voluntary sector, in a way that takes no account of the kind of health care provision that nurses themselves might prefer. Any opposition is easily overcome once these large-scale ideological shifts have become established and come to appear the natural way to deliver health care.

The notion of ideology, then, helps to explain the phenomenon whereby people are pressured into acting in broadly similar ways and sometimes accepting new philosophies unquestioningly. It also helps to explain why people sometimes act in ways that are not in their immediate interests. The notion of ideology has, however, been challenged as an oversimplification (Henriques *et al.*, 1984).

The traditional notion of ideology appears to be in need of modification if the huge range of thinking on every issue which is so evident in society today is to be taken into account. It is difficult to argue that we are all involved in the reproduction of a single dominant ideology when contemporary life is characterized by disagreement and diversity. Nurses who work in hospitals do not necessarily live out a medical ideology in their private lives, but may be avid experimenters with alternative therapies. A nurse who appears for work at a hospital wearing her Animal Liberation Front badge may be told by her manager to take it off because it is inappropriate to bring politics into the workplace. Yet, at the same time, the UK health service is being transformed by constant politically led changes in the NHS – so clearly *some* kinds of politics are allowed. The point is that it is difficult to think of human social life as being propelled by a single ideology and there are many contradictions and inconsistencies (Billig *et al.*, 1987).

Nurses need to grapple with the notion of ideology because it helps explain how language may be instrumental in propping up outdated and inappropriate working practices. It reveals how language is embedded in and inseparable from the social context. Most importantly, it highlights the fact that systems of ideas are only ever partial and can never quite address every individual's personal situation.

NURSING AND POSTMODERNISM

Spoken and written communication is a vital aspect of nursing activity, not least in handing over care to colleagues and recording the delivery of care in a wide variety of documentation. Recently, the demand for nurses to communicate effectively in both speech and writing has become more important as a wide audience of patients, purchasers, professional bodies and the law demand satisfaction. However, research has only recently begun to focus on language in the nursing literature. Because this fundamental concern has not been sufficiently emphasized, language has been frequently used by nurses in an unthinking manner. This artlessness has been revealed in a lack of awareness of the way in which words impact upon care and has left nurses ill-equipped to define exactly what they mean in the language they use.

For anyone to define exactly what they mean in the language they use is, of course, no easy matter. A huge academic industry has grown up around the question of language, trying to establish what language does, how it can achieve meaning, whether it mirrors or creates reality, to what extent human beings and their cultures are constructed by language, how powerful it is, how ideological it is. Disciplines as diverse as philosophy, linguistics, anthropology, literary criticism, psychology and sociology have tackled the problem of language and meaning.

An increased scepticism about accepted values and a greater willingness to question what has gone before, or what anything means, is at the centre of what is known as 'postmodernism'. This term cuts across so many different academic disciplines and points of view that it is often seen as a difficult and confusing concept. However, it is a concept that theorists of nursing are increasingly turning to as a way of making sense of the late twentieth-century experience of health care. Therefore, to make sense of its appeal to nursing scholars, let us explore the background to this term in a little more detail.

'Postmodernism', the 'postmodern' and 'postmodernity' are generally thought to concern artistic, cultural and social changes that followed the massive trauma and chaos of the Second World War. Following this war, traditional notions of truth, reason and ultimate explanations were left in tatters. A depthless, playful and questioning mood invaded cultural, artistic and social aspects of life, from art, architecture, literature and film to notions of the human condition or society's sense of itself. This scepticism was the culmination of a growing dissatisfaction with the ability of science, technology and reason to improve the human condition. It called into doubt the progress of modernity from the sudden enthusiasm for science in the eighteenth-century Enlightenment through to the present day.

Hans Bertens (1995) offers a refreshingly comprehensive and readable account of the history of postmodernism. 'Postmodernism,' he writes, 'is several things at once. It refers, first of all, to a complex of anti-modernist artistic strategies which emerged in the 1950s and developed momentum in the course of the 1960s' (p. 3), became involved with the poststructuralist debate in the 1970s concerning 'representations that do not represent' (p. 7), and grew more politicized in the 1980s as a 'postmodernism' that 'attempts to expose the

Key reference

politics that are at work in representations and to undo institutional-ised hierarchies' and counter these by advocating 'difference, pluriformity, and multiplicity' (p. 8). This advocacy of 'difference' was at the hub of feminism and multiculturalism, which gained momentum in the 1980s and involved a strong interest in minority points of view and marginalized voices. 'Postmodernism,' Bertens writes, is a 'perspective from which [the] world is seen' (p. 9) and has moved out from the field of humanities into all other disciplines of inquiry. Bertens attempts to encapsulate what is at the heart of 'postmodernism' or, rather, the various 'postmodernisms' that have presented themselves in the second half of the twentieth century:

> If there is a common denominator to all these postmodernisms, it is that of a crisis in representation: a deeply felt loss of faith in our ability to represent the real, in the widest sense. No matter whether they are aesthetic, epistemological, moral, or political in nature, the representations that we used to rely on can no longer be taken for granted. Whatever its origins, which are diagnosed in different ways by Daniel Bell, Lyotard, Jameson, and other theorists, this crisis in representation has far-reaching consequences. Some would seem to be debilitating. For example, now that transcendent truth seems forever out of reach, hermeneutics must replace our former aspirations to objectivity . . . Other consequences are positively enabling. If all representations are constructs that ultimately are politically informed, then it should be possible, for instance, to break away from our current ones.
> (p. 11)

In health care, there is now a growing emphasis on evidence-based practice and reflection, but applying postmodern thinking to health care means we have to question what is meant by evidence and practice. Ideas about what constitutes evidence and practice themselves may be controversial. There are a multitude of ways in which nursing activities may be understood, described, justified or disseminated. Often, a variety of ideas are in competition with each other and will not result in any clear-cut pathways for care. The diversity becomes clear as soon as we consider how many kinds of nursing intervention are available. There may be, for example, competition between biomedical and psychosocial interventions. Nurses may argue for different treatment regimes in wound care or for different counselling approaches. Some nurses may prefer working closely with families of clients; others may see this as ineffectual, unhelpful or intrusive. The list, of course, is endless and always growing as new interventions, strategies or models emerge.

Whether it wants to be or not, nursing finds itself in the postwar maelstrom of postmodernism, which offers opportunities for analysing more critically the accepted versions of what nursing is and can become. Some may prefer to view the uncertain diversity of nursing as 'debilitating' or as a threat to its foundations and to respond by advocating a larger dose of objectivity and standardization in the profession. Others might find it 'enabling' because calling into question the old certainties and models of what nursing achieves might yield new and better foundations. This book stands somewhere between dystopian fears about postmodern uncertainty and utopian claims for the liberation and freedom that postmodernism brings. Some may argue that this is just sitting on the fence. We would argue that this third position or 'excluded middle' is the *latest* postmodernism. We consider that a postmodern critique of nursing foundations, and, in this book, its language, does not have to bring the dizzying sense that 'nothing is certain' or 'everything is relative'. Rather, it can both have a sobering effect on those who are too dogmatic about what nursing is and does and also avoid playing into the hands of crisis mongers and relativists who want to destroy its foundations in the name of liberty. We scrutinize nursing language not to proclaim its demise or celebrate a crisis in the meaning of nursing, but to inspire its renaissance. Such a renaissance would involve an increasing number of nurses becoming critically aware of the power and politics of language in health care. Some grasp of postmodernism is vital if nurses are to see the limitations and possibilities for any future nursing language.

In part, postmodernism is to do with increasing scepticism about the ability of 'grand narratives' – or big stories – to explain and improve the human condition. The grand narratives that have held such sway in the past include the assumption that science and technology would automatically yield better ways of living (no longer tenable in the face of diminishing world resources, global warming and pollution) and the theories of Marxism and psychoanalysis which sought to explain the human condition. In medicine and nursing there is a growing feeling that much of what is done in the name of treatment may be ineffective, expensive and sometimes harmful. In the UK, it could be argued that what has happened to the health service with its fragmentation into purchasers, providers and fund holders and the loss of a coherent institutional framework is a prime example of postmodernism.

More generally, we now live in a world of hyper-communication. The new information technology churns out vast amounts of texts and images that bombard us with different versions of reality. Indeed, thinkers such as Jacques Derrida (1976) have cast considerable doubt over any possibility of representing the world exhaustively and accurately. Thus, postmodernism prioritizes language as a major feature of social life, and insists that meanings are not defined by their correspondence with an external reality but that they have to be seen and qualified within their social contexts. Because contexts are so variable it is difficult to make any definite statements about the world in general. Broadly then, a postmodernist view emphasizes discourse or 'language in use' as the thing that constitutes reality. We will say more on the problems of language representing the world in chapter 4.

So far, we have described postmodernism as if it were something radically new, but it may be seen as having continuity with modernity, as Scanell, Schlesinger and Sparks (1992) write: 'Whether postmodernism represents a sharp break from modernity or simply a late stage in that historical development is the crux of the matter' (p. 2). Perhaps the radical scepticism of postmodernism is derived from the familiar scientific scepticism of the Enlightenment. It could be that this reflexive concern with evidence and the foundations of knowledge has led to the uncertainty that pervades postmodernism. As Bertens (1995, p. 247) argues, 'the self-reflexivity inherent in the modern project has come to question modernity at large. In the last twenty years, modernity, as a grand socio-political project, has increasingly been called to account by itself; modernity has turned its critical rationality upon itself and has been forced to reluctantly admit to its costs.' In other words, the desire for evidence, explanations and certainty about the world has yielded an increasingly sceptical attitude among scientists and within intellectual life at large. This suggests that a certain amount of continuity exists between modernism and postmodernism.

On the other hand, a discontinuity between modernism – the Enlightenment quest for rational explanations and knowledge – and postmodernism is often central to the definition of the latter: 'Modernism acknowledged the fragmentary, transient, dislocated character of the social world but tried to overcome it, to retrieve a lost unity, whereas postmodernism is content to accept and celebrate a de-centred political, economic and cultural global environment. It rejects deep structures, any notion of an underlying, determining reality. It accepts a world of appearances, a surface reality without depth' (Scannell, Schlesinger and Sparks, 1992, p. 3).

In terms of health care, one way of thinking about the contrast between modernism and postmodernism is to consider different approaches to making sense of illness. A modernist ambition might be to try to find out what the patient's real problem is and to do this by the use of stethoscopes, blood tests, CAT scans and diagnostic interviews. The idea is that, however incoherent the patient's symptoms, there must be some unitary underlying pathology which can be discovered by the skilled clinician. From a postmodernist perspective, the patient's anxiety about who will feed her cat, or look after her children, is as much a feature of her illness experience as the swelling, fracture or blood test results. More seriously, many critics of health care have foregrounded the fact that patients often feel oppressed, let down or even abused by health care systems that were ostensibly put in place to help them. Postmodernism invites us to address these marginalized voices or positions. Later in this book we will be exploring these perspectives further.

If we take postmodernist thinking at face value, there are disturbing implications for the practice of health care (Clarke, 1996). If it is impossible for nurses to reach a satisfactory understanding of what they do, if reality is indeed indeterminate, this calls into question the value of their work. Equally, researchers cannot be sure that the data they have so painstakingly gathered will be sufficiently convincing or significant. Nonetheless, there are some important opportunities that come with the postmodernist assault on convention. It can sensitize us to the fact that there may be conflicting opinions about illness, which will be different for doctors, nurses, the patient, the acupuncturist or the homeopath, for example. Postmodernism allows us to grasp this diverse picture without feeling the need to establish 'the truth'. Some may find such diversity in health care approaches 'debilitating' while others find it 'enabling'. Nurses who find diverse and often conflicting accounts of illness and health care debilitating may attempt to exclude significant interpretations and apply narrow strategies of care. We argue in the course of this book that nurses should pay closer attention to the diverse nature of health care interventions. We believe that diversity should be welcomed and explored in the hope that this will lead to more flexible, effective and compassionate interventions. In other words, an appreciation of diversity by nurses may enable them to interpret better the realities of the people they care for.

LANGUAGE IN ACTION

Despite the pervading sense in postmodernism that language is incapable of representing reality, many theorists have tried to arrive at plausible interpretations of what words can do and mean. The speech act theory of Austin (1962), Searle (1969) and Grice (1975) has been useful in this regard – examining how actions are performed through speech. Recent developments in analysing conversation and discourse show up some fundamental problems in medical and nursing knowledge. By thinking carefully about what is said in the course of conversation, it can be seen that speakers are not simply conversing about events or environments, but are mutually constructing them. Discourse analysis draws attention to the way in which health care language produces the sense that carers are talking about a world that is external to their patients.

In much analysis of the nature of language, there is a tendency for the written text to be considered more highly than the spoken word. For example, in grammar, what we call the 'parts of speech' are usually based on the language as it is written. In health care situations too, the fact that written records are permanent and that they are very important if legal issues arise or patients complain mean that they are often given a higher status than what has been said. The written language of nursing can be analysed in reports, care plans and patients' notes and it is easy to see how verbal communications between nurses, nursing students, doctors, social workers and other staff are informed by the linguistic structure of written records.

It is not, perhaps, immediately apparent that what nurses say in spoken or written texts can be actions as well as records. When a nurse, for example, orders a patient to stop doing something, the effect of her words may well be that the patient does indeed stop. Here the words: 'Stop that!' can be seen to have a similar power to the act of physically stopping someone from doing something. Equally, the way that a nurse judges a person in written and spoken text may well act against the person in a very obvious way. She may communicate that a client is 'manipulative' and this negative tag then affects how that client feels about himself if it is said directly to him, or the way in which others respond to him if such a meaning is conveyed in spoken or written reports to others. Such negative communicative acts are far from the ideal of promoting well- being. Since nurses perform a variety of speech acts in their daily work, it is clearly important to examine them critically.

We know that language can *do* things or act upon people. We perhaps take for granted how we shape the world around us with language. Requests, commands, promises and threats are examples of the way in which different kinds of language affect us quite differently. The capacity to disrupt or change the course of history by such simple commands as 'No! Don't do that!' or 'That's fine, carry on!' go unnoticed. Every time we open our mouths or put pen to paper, we take a political and moral stance towards the future. The care people often take when writing letters is a reminder of the seriousness of words. Often they will draft and redraft letters, knowing that what they write will be interpreted at a distance, without the chance for them to say 'No, I didn't mean it quite like that' or 'That isn't what I said'. Here, there is a recognition that the written word can easily be misinterpreted. The same unease can apply to spoken language. For example, most of us will be aware of how we try to edit the words we say before they leave our mouths when attending a job interview. Equally, we can acknowledge the seriousness of reading and listening to other people's communications. We tend to examine closely a written contract before signing it, or to listen attentively when a tutor gives indications of what to expect in an examination. In these examples, not to pay close attention to words could have unwelcome consequences. Since we write, speak, read and listen carefully in many different ways in everyday life, and have an awareness of the possible consequences of our failure to do so, it is only right to examine the status of nursing communications that carry great responsibility for the futures of others.

The potential damage of nursing communication lies not simply in what nurses speak and write, but also in the way in which they receive other people's spoken and written words. In terms of the perils of speaking we might think of the graphic research of Thomas *et al.* (1984) and Garvin *et al.* (1992), who found that a patient's heart rate and blood pressure can be affected by what is said to him and advised that nurses should be particularly sensitive to the potentially harmful impact of their words and those of visiting relatives upon cardiac patients. In writing, we should be concerned, for example, about how nurses represent those in their care and linguistically incarcerate them by using judgemental words and phrases and even citing false information. By listening to unethical statements about those in our care and not doing anything to counter such statements is not to listen at all. Rather, it is to permit potential damage or harm to those for whom we stand as advocates. Finally, to read objectionable, libellous or defamatory accounts of individuals and not take action to rectify such linguistic crimes is to step down from the responsibilities of caring for others. Yet critical listening and reading does not simply mean that nurses should monitor their own speech and writing, but, importantly, that they should scrutinize the speech and writing produced by other health care professionals such as doctors, psychologists, social workers and so on. By first reflecting critically on their own language, nurses may gain the right, and indeed the skills, to challenge the language of others.

Diversity in the meanings that can be assigned to language adds up to a 'strain' on the use of language. Nurses need to be aware of this strain; the words they speak or write may convey meanings they did not anticipate or desire. Although nurses, like everyone else, can never guarantee the meanings of their spoken or written words, they need to reduce the scope for misinterpretation and remain vigilant when considering the meanings of other people's spoken and written texts. The strain on meaning in language combined with the power of language to construct the world in which we live make it more important than ever for nurses to monitor health care language as it affects the lives of others. To pay attention to what is spoken and written about the people that nurses care for is vital if nursing is to continue its tradition of advocacy. If nurses have no critical interest in how they talk to and write about those in their care, or how patients give account of themselves, or how other professionals describe them, then they no longer deserve to be thought of as practising nurses. Effectively, nurses who do not communicate *carefully* are not caring.

THE TEXTUALITY OF NURSING

Communication in nursing can take place with spoken and written language, and also with the use of images and signs. All these forms of communication can be classed as texts in nursing care. Nursing practice is constructed by a variety of texts, such as procedure manuals, nursing policy documents, videos of nursing procedures, diagrams of techniques and the nursing process itself, which forms a kind of backbone to nursing language. The language of nursing is clearly dominated by the language of medicine and science, threatened by the possibility of legal action, and struggling to represent its own philosophy and dogma. The construction of nursing along the lines of being 'caring' or 'nurturing' remains subordinate to the dominant construction of medicine as scientific (Cheek and Rudge, 1994). For this hierarchy to be challenged, or more realistically mitigated, nurses need to become more critically aware of how health care language is constructed to keep them in their place. Levine (1989) suggests that the way forward is not by continuing the conflict between those who support a nursing or a medical diagnosis, but by bringing about a 'joint effort to find clinical diagnostic language of universal meaning to clinical practitioners in all health care professions' (p. 5). This kind of reductionism, however, runs the risk of losing many of the features that are unique to each health care specialism.

It is unlikely that the talk and writing that nurses engage in will topple or shout louder than the talk and writing of medicine. The scientific discourse of the latter forms almost the last of the grand narratives mentioned earlier in this chapter which incorporate and attempt to give meaning to a whole range of bodily and mental phenomena. For the moment, this medical and scientific system of thought will continue explaining, supervising and regulating the bodies of patients and staff alike. Nurses should choose instead to emphasize their role in acting as advocates for patients' interests, and to offer alternatives to the medical discourses. Opportunities arise when they write in patients' records, when they talk informally in common rooms and offices, when they write letters to nursing magazines and participate in management consultation exercises. If the actual practice of nursing really is reflected by the way in which it is communicated, then the greatest opportunity for nursing to become truly holistic is to maximize its own language, in competition with the other languages found in the workplace, such as the languages of medicine and management. As a competing language, we might refer to it as an 'anti-language'. This is because we propose that nursing language can undermine the dominant discourses of medicine or financial management to the benefit of nurses and patients. In essence, nursing language can be a site of resistance to the medical and economic discourses that currently dominate modern health care. Walker (1995) suggests that nurses need to define or redefine their culture by means of the words they use, oral and written, in both clinical and research practice.

RECORD KEEPING

Many texts in the education of nurses influence how they communicate. Written communication, in particular, is dictated by the nursing process of assessment, planning, implementation and evaluation. Despite having this framework, documentation is often problematic for nurses: 'However it is named in its endless variety of forms, both the process and the product of writing about care have proven to be unsatisfactory for practising nurses' (Hays, 1989, p. 200). Nurses have to write under numerous constraints. In translating care into text, nurses may often feel as if they have to walk through a minefield of potential criticism. Not only are they under pressure to record those nursing interventions that can easily be costed, but they must also adhere to the UKCC's *Standards for Records and Record Keeping*:

> **The following principles must apply: the record is directed primarily to serving the interests of the patient or client to whom it relates and enabling the provision of care, the prevention of disease and the promotion of health; the record demonstrates the accurate chronology of events and all significant consultations, assessments, observations, decisions, interventions and outcomes;**

the record and the activity of record keeping is an integral and essential part of care and not a distraction from its provision; the record is clear and unambiguous; the record contains entries recording facts and observations written at the time of, or soon after, the events described; the record provides a safe and effective means of communication between members of the health care team and supports continuity of care; the record demonstrates that the practitioner's duty of care has been fulfilled; the systems for record keeping exclude unauthorised access and breaches of confidentiality and the record is constructed and completed in such a manner as to facilitate the monitoring of standards, audit, quality assurance and the investigation of complaints.

(UKCC, 1993, p. 16)

The UKCC includes directions for how entries in patients' records are to be physically made:

Records must: be written legibly and indelibly; be clear and unambiguous; be accurate in each entry as to date and time; ensure that alterations are made by scoring out with a single line followed by the initialed, dated and timed correct entry; ensure that additions to existing entries are individually dated, timed and signed; not include abbreviations, meaningless phrases and offensive subjective statements unrelated to the patient's care and associated observations; not allow the use of initials for major entries and, where their use is allowed for other entries, ensure that local arrangements for identifying initials and signatures exist and not include entries made in pencil or blue ink, the former carrying the risk of erasure and the latter (where photocopying is required) of poor quality reproduction. (pp. 6–7)

Almost lost in this morass of guidelines about such things as which pen to choose is the statement that nurses should not include abbreviations, meaningless phrases and offensive subjective statements unrelated to the patient's care and associated observations. The UKCC hopes, no doubt, that meaningless phrases and offensive subjective statements are as easily controlled as the colour of ink used for writing patients' records. But *how exactly* are nurses to avoid being meaningless or offensive? How are records to be made clear and unambiguous? Such issues deserve a UKCC publication all of their own!

Nurses must write with the knowledge that patients, colleagues and lawyers might want to read what they have written. They are required to describe briefly, using the template of the nursing process, what can be very complex nursing interventions. Armed with a black pen and a whole protocol for how to sign and date their entries, the nurse must become a responsible author. No wonder, perhaps, that nurses avoid writing anything but what they think to be safe. As Levine (1989) argues, nursing language frequently says nothing at all:

While in part it is a reflection of an inadequate education in the liberal arts and humanities, historically nurses have been in

> conflict when they were required to understand, but not use freely, a precise language vital to nursing practice. Nurses interpreted and used with skill and insight the information conveyed by the language of medical diagnosis. But there was always a game that had to be played. Nothing was ever certain. The nurse recorded only things that 'seemed' to be or described with requisite uncertainty 'apparent' observations. A haemorrhage was 'bright, red drainage' because the correct term was a diagnosis; and yet the nurse knew when the alarm needed to be sounded . . . Charged with the conviction that they needed to record *something* about the patient's activities, they quickly learned how to say nothing with elegance: 'Slept well'; 'Good appetite'; 'Up and about'; 'No complaints'; 'Resting comfortably.' Nurses found many ways to say nothing in situations where they believed there was nothing to say, that is, where no obvious interventions were necessary. Everyone knew that they were slogans and that little faith was invested in what nurses reported and recorded in the nurse's notes. (p. 5)

The challenge, as Levine (1989) sees it, is for nurses 'to talk about what they do in language that clearly states the nature of their work . . . To nurse ethically, we must say what we mean and always mean what we say' (p. 6). Hays (1989) believes that despite the powerful constraints operating on nursing language, nurses can learn to do justice to care in text:

> Most nurses, at least those who endure, thrive on the nurse–patient encounter with all its unpredictability and peril; this should give us hope for the secondary activity: the translation of care into words. If we can achieve excellence in increasingly complex patient care, we can learn to describe it in words. However, writing about care must be taught not as a poor step-sister to nursing care itself, but as a primary activity of the discipline along with physical assessment, patient advocacy, ethical decision making and sterile technique. (p. 203)

Such learning, Hays suggests, must include an awareness of nursing discourse as a political and moral undertaking in conflict with other discourses. A balance needs to be struck between unconstrained writing and writing that is constrained by culture, profession and tradition. In order to do this, she recommends that: (a) nurses identify constraints and their underlying values and examine how it is that they 'make themselves heard in the record' (p. 203); (b) look at how care activities are described; (c) attempt descriptions from different perspectives and engage the patient in documentation.

Narratives

The storytelling aspect of nursing language is generally overlooked. Much of our communication with others is in the form of storytelling.

We tell stories about ourselves and our place in the world or about others and their place in the world. We interpret people's narrations of themselves and others. To date, nurses have had little opportunity to study how much of their work depends on the stories they tell about themselves and about those for whom they care. Nurses narrate both their own stories of care and the stories told to them by patients. This doesn't mean that the stories nurses tell are pure fictions. What it does mean is that much of what happens between nurses and patients is to do with narration. This idea has been developed in psychology, sociology, anthropology and in the study of medical and nursing activities and the experiences of patients.

What is a narrative?

The concern with narratives emerges from the everyday observation that when we find out about someone we usually do so by means of a story which they tell or which someone else tells about them. As Riessman (1993) puts it, 'Nature and the world do not tell stories; individuals do. Interpretation is inevitable because narratives are representations' (p. 2). These stories are important because they do not merely describe experience but constitute it (Ricouer, 1991):

> How individuals recount their histories, what they emphasise and omit, their stance as protagonists or victims, the relationship the story establishes between the teller and audience – all shape what individuals can claim of their own lives. Personal stories are not merely a way of telling someone (or oneself) about one's life, they are the means by which identities may be fashioned.
>
> *(Rosenwald and Ochberg, 1992, p. 1)*

Labov (1972; 1982; Labov and Waletzky, 1967) argues that most fully formed narratives have six major aspects, namely: (1) an abstract – that is a brief overview of the story; (2) orientation – setting the scene, time and place; (3) complicating action – this is what makes the events into a story or disrupts the equilibrium; (4) evaluation – where decisions are taken and actions are entered into; (5) resolution – where the actions either do or do not have the desired effect; and (6) coda – sometimes in the form of a moral or short phrase that sums the story up. In a similar way, Burke (1945) categorizes act, scene, agent, agency and purpose and claims that several or all of these are present in an intelligible linguistic sequence.

Narratives reflect the interest of the teller. Hyden (1992) describes how, in cases of domestic violence, male perpetrators favour words that emphasize purpose (why they acted as they did) whereas wives emphasize agency (how they were beaten) and the physical and emotional consequences (Lempert, 1994). Bruner (1984) says, 'A life as told, a life history, is a narrative, influenced by the cultural conventions of telling, by the audience, and by the social context' (p. 7).

Denzin (1989) believes that biographies have a tendency to freeze lived events into rigid sequences and this tendency is even more evident when the story is written up by analysts. Denzin believes that people's stories often become transformed into 'epiphanies', that is manifestations or interactional moments that alter the fundamental meaning structure in a person's life. They represent a threshold between one way of telling the self and another.

Truths may be layered; they may be presented at one time in a certain way only to be revised later. For example, Denzin describes an Alcoholics Anonymous member who disclosed that he had in fact been drinking during the time he had been claiming to be sober. Conventionally, we would say that the first version was 'lies' and the second version was 'truth'. This misses the point. First, the earlier version was presented and accepted as a truth at the time, and second, the later version may well be revised itself on a later occasion. In best postmodernist tradition, the truth itself is never fully resolved. Narrative analysis offers possibilities for linking the author's experience to the enterprise of social science. This is particularly clear when it comes to accounts of illness.

Narrating illness

Our most fundamental ideas about medicine are embedded in culture and language. In the UK in the 1990s, most people would think that they know what a sick person is. However, history suggests that the way illness is defined today depends a great deal on fairly recent changes in patterns of sickness and health:

> The appearance of today's 'sick person' seems predicated on at least three conditions: first, disease must cease to be a mass phenomenon [e.g. plagues and epidemics]; second, illness must not be followed immediately by death; and third, it is probably also necessary that the diversity of suffering be reduced by a unifying general view which is precisely that of clinical medicine.
>
> (Herzlich and Pierret, 1987, p. 23)

In the late twentieth century, everyday complaints like the common cold and gastrointestinal upsets have a set of symptoms that we expect to co-occur. As sufferers or healers, we tend to look for distinct patterns in illness. The illnesses we identify are different from those described in the eighteenth century – we no longer claim to suffer from 'seizures of the bowels' or 'rising of the lights'. Nevertheless, in all centuries, the coherence of an illness is an important part of the sufferer's experience of it.

Consistency in illness

Let us consider the narrative quoted by Charnaz (1991; 1995) of a woman suffering from systemic lupus erythematosus, a disorder of the connective tissues, primarily affecting women in their thirties and forties. It may involve arthritis, and problems with the kidneys, heart and brain.

> If you have lupus, I mean one day it's my liver; one day it's my joints; one day it's my head, and it's like people really think you're

a hypochondriac if you keep complaining about different ailments
. . . It's like you don't want to say anything because people are
going to start thinking, you know, 'God, don't go near her, all she
is . . . is complaining about this.' And I think that's why I never
say anything because I feel like everything I have is related one
way or another to the lupus but most of the people don't know I
have lupus, and even those that do are not going to believe that
ten different ailments are the same thing. And I don't want
anybody saying, you know, [that] they don't want to come around
me because I complain. (pp. 114–15)

This kind of description is often inaccessible in ordinary discourse,
says Charnaz, because etiquette and social convention limit disclosures
of illness. However, in circumstances where such accounts can be
produced, we immediately see the important role narratives play in
making sense of the illness experience and the problems that ensue
when it does not easily fit with what the narrator sees to be the ideas
of illness that other people are working with.

What may also become apparent from patients' narratives is how
people have changed as a result of becoming ill. Frank (1993) notes
that there are a great many academic and popular accounts of self
change. As one commentator declared in the case of HIV, 'Our new
date of birth is the day when we discovered that we carried AIDS
inside us' (Dreuilhe, 1988, p. 151). May (1991) describes the case of
a man who was severely burned and who changed his name to 'Dax'.
This was partly because he needed a name that could be written easily
with his reconstructed hands but also because he wished to declare
that his new post-burn self was different from the previous person he
had been. May draws an analogy with the Phoenix: 'If the patient
revives after such events, he must reconstruct afresh, tap new power,
and appropriate patterns that help define a new existence. One cannot
talk simply of a new accessory [prosthesis] here, a change of venue
there, but . . . of a new Phoenix that must emerge from the ashes'
(p. 22). However, the analogy with the Phoenix is not entirely apt, as
May goes on to describe: 'The Phoenix remembers nothing of its
former life. The burn victim, however, remembers his past. The
persistence of memory establishes continuity with the past but also
reinforces his sense of distance from it' (p. 26).

In a study of individuals with cancer diagnoses by Mathieson and
Stam (1995), people reported that they were increasingly understood
by others, especially medical staff, in terms of their illness rather than
as individuals. One woman described how she was told by a doctor
about the progress of her illness:

Key reference

He came in, and I'm in a quad room – four people – there's a few
nurses around, a couple of cleaning ladies . . . Some people had
company and he didn't even pull the curtains around my bed to
tell me I had recurring cancer, and that I had a tumour the size
of the hand, and that it was total removal if this [further treatment]
was unsuccessful. Everybody was staring at me . . . I was just

> devastated . . . and he came back to me the next day and he said
> 'I'm really sorry I did that', and I said, 'Well, I know you must
> have a lot on your mind but the offence here is that you see me
> as a tumour, not as a person'. (pp. 295–6)

The problem for the patient with this transformed identity is com-
pounded not only by the response of health care professionals but by
the reactions of others:

> I couldn't have run out to my four best friends and said 'I got it
> girls, I got the Big C' . . . I travel in a group of women, and one
> of these women had serious cancer, and I saw her the other day
> . . . and I looked at her and I thought . . . I couldn't think anything
> else of her, I couldn't think what a fabulous person she was, I
> mean, she had in capital letters, written from the top of her head
> to the bottom of her shoe, CANCER, and I couldn't get beyond
> that to see the person she was.
>
> *(Mathieson and Stam, 1995, p. 297)*

Some participants in Mathieson's and Stam's study reported dramatic
withdrawals from friendships. Even after the active phase of cancer
treatment was over, people continued renegotiating their identity to
incorporate their sense of stigma. It is just this kind of dominating
storyline which nurses read into the faces of those they care for. It
takes extra-special effort to resist the monologue of illness and explore
other narrations. Not seeing the damaging effects of the illness story
will deprive nurses of opportunities to understand the multi-storied
person.

In some kinds of illness, such as stroke, the patient's ability to tell
a coherent story may be reduced and the piecing together of stories
more laboured. In a study by Manzo, Blonder and Burns (1995), the
researchers noted how male stroke patients were assisted by their
wives in formulating the story of their illness. The patients often
sought approval from their spouses for what they were trying to say,
asking tag questions such as 'Didn't I?' and 'Isn't that right?' The
spouse sometimes answered questions directed at the patient on his
behalf – this tendency was so compelling that the researchers found
themselves interviewing the spouse rather than the patient. In addition, spouses sometimes engaged in competitive storytelling, supple-
menting or contradicting the story told by the patient. In the following
brief example from the research of Manzo, Blonder and Burns (1995,
p. 315), 'I' is the interviewer, 'H' is the husband and 'W' is the wife.

I: This is May 5, 1988. I'd like to begin by just asking you if you can
describe how you knew you had a stroke and what happened, what
were the symptoms and did you g–, when did you go to the hospital,
things like that?

H: Well, I went in, ah: oh, November, right? (*to wife*)

W: September.

H: September.

W: Friday the 13th.

H: Ah, down here, and then a – after a couple of weeks they figured I was to go to the Veterans' Hospital.

This extract demonstrates how the business of telling the story of illness may be a joint production, with the details reconstructed by two or more people. The authors point out that this aspect of social support after a stroke has both advantages and disadvantages: 'In the short term, it seems unquestionably true, and makes good sense, that the presence of a significant other is important for stroke patients' post-stroke rehabilitation. In the longer term, however, this blessing can become a curse' (p. 323). The joint telling of stories may go against the patient regaining independence and language skills of his own. Nurses working with stroke victims or those with other brain disorders that disrupt language need to remain alert to this aspect of narration. Wherever possible, they need to encourage communication by the affected persons themselves, and to be careful in interpreting information from significant others such as spouses.

In a study by Yoshida (1993) of people with severe spinal injuries, disability altered the consciousness of respondents in numerous ways. One spoke of how he was now conscious of the way in which able-bodied society deals with people who are disabled:

Mr MK: If someone comes by wanting to help me, I would tell them, 'Thank you very much, but I don't need it. I can probably handle it, but I appreciate your help.' Because, who knows? The next guy down the road might not be so lucky. To be able to do it himself. He might get stuck one day. And if I yell at him, the guy here, he will go down the street and he will see the other guy and say, 'Oh well, I won't touch you. Go ahead, help yourself.' And I don't think that is fair. (p. 230)

Different respondents narrated their disability in different ways. Thus one informant said that he had become aware that requiring assistance aligned him with other groups in society:

Mr GS: I would like to see a more aware world for physically disabled people. But I don't want to see a [totally] accessible one. I want to see people being helped into and helped out and it becomes an accepted thing . . . When somebody is crossing the street, when you see an older person crossing the street and the cars start to go, somebody runs out and says, 'Stop! This lady is still crossing the street.' (p. 230)

Using different scenarios to tell a coherent story about one's situation is a vital part of making sense of the situation to oneself, the researcher and presumably to friends, family and colleagues. It is also a way of locating oneself in relation to others. We do not simply make comparisons between ourselves and other people, but we include actual or hypothetical people in stories to establish identity and difference.

So narratives are important in establishing the individual's experience and identity in relation to those of others and in making sense of illness and health. Examining the stories patients tell can yield insights into the processes that modify or maintain the illness or even make the situation better. This storied nature of experience is fundamental to medical anthropology (Kleinman, 1988; Good, 1990). It is vital for nurses to recognize just how much of what they do is concerned with storytelling.

Researchers have studied the narratives that attach to human lives as a whole, to episodes of illness and being told one is ill, but most research treats the narratives as if they were texts which the researcher can simply examine for themes, features or structure. The assumption is that the real business of being ill or being treated happens somewhere else or at another time, and the story is merely retold when the researcher switches on a tape recorder. This assumption is misleading because it fails to take into account how stories are told and retold in care settings from moment to moment.

A new departure in narrative analysis is to accept that each care encounter has a narrative of its own. From the point of view of the client, going to the doctor's, a session of occupational therapy or being visited by a health visitor each has its own plot. This has been explored by Mattingly (1994), who writes, 'Clinical encounters involve clinician and patient in the creation and negotiation of a plot structure within clinical time' (p. 811).

Mattingly describes occupational therapy with a patient who has suffered a head injury and who awoke from a coma a few days earlier. She shows how the therapist encourages the patient to comb his hair, saying that it is good for learning balance. However, when the hair-combing session is over, another kind of plot seems to have developed. The patient indicates that he wants a mirror, which the therapist provides. So as well as being a medical procedure to improve balance, the hair-combing session develops a self-care theme. The occupational therapist then says in a jocular way, 'Going to make yourself look good for your girlfriend?' Although this piece of talk is laden with heterosexist assumptions about why people modify their appearance, it is also a way of making the action meaningful.

There may be larger-scale plots at work in the therapeutic encounter, such as the strongly held assumption that, if we are ill, going to the doctor will make us better, or at least set the process of healing in motion. Both lay people and professionals assume that health care involves description and diagnosis of the problem and some sort of therapy or treatment with consequent abatement of the symptoms. Patients and staff work together to sustain these therapeutic plots or narratives.

DISCIPLINES OF CARE, DISCIPLINES OF LANGUAGE

As health professionals are educated and trained in separate groups, they are encouraged to think of their own discipline as being distinct from other disciplines. Occupational therapists' sense of themselves is different from nurses' and social workers'. Children's nurses want to distinguish themselves from coronary care nurses or midwives. Mental health nurses in community care are quick to describe how their work differs from the work of hospital-based nurse work, perhaps in terms of how the old-style hospital psychiatry was dominated by medical assumptions, whereas they are concerned to empower the clients and mobilize their own support system.

These distinct identities encourage a view that the practice of care is highly differentiated. However, there are some social and linguistic processes that occur in a variety of health care contexts. The judgements made by professionals may slip across disciplines, as is apparent in areas such as mental health, where people's complex living problems are easily reinterpreted. On the other hand, broken bones and burst appendices are, it might be argued, rather different. Here, the problem is clear-cut, and the solution equally straightforward.

Such a claim ignores the diversity of healing practices around the world and throughout history. It is conventional to claim that other kinds of medicine are but pale imitations of western medicine. They may contain a grain of truth, but they are largely based on superstition, unlike the scientific practices of health care professionals in Europe and North America. However, it is vital to see other ways of healing for what they are – integrated social systems which are carried on by people every bit as sophisticated as westerners.

Secondly, there is evidence that even scientific medicine may allow non-scientific considerations to creep in. Hunt, Litt and Loebner (1988) report a study of adolescent women admitted to hospital in the USA with abdominal pains. If the woman was black or Hispanic, and especially if she was working class, she was much more likely to be asked questions about heterosexual sex experiences, contraceptive use and possible pregnancy than were her white, middle-class peers. It is possible to explain this clinical scrutiny of the sex lives of young women of colour in the USA as indicative of the concerns of white academic and political elites about the development of an underclass in US society. Large-scale political concerns may be represented at the level of the clinical encounter.

Thirdly, there are inequalities in decision-making power in medicine. Consider, for example, the level of control that women have over their own fertility. As Griffin (1992) argues, it is becoming increasingly difficult for women to obtain an abortion. However, the picture is 'very different for young women who want to give birth, especially if they are living outside, or on the margins of the affluent First World', and if they are likely to be constructed as 'irresponsible mothers' (p. 492).

In such cases, their fate may well be sterilization in the form of genetic counselling, sterilization without consent during gynaecological operations, or even being paid to be sterilized under a World Health Organisation scheme. Thus, clinical judgements are often intertwined with issues of power and politics. In the case of abortion, the rhetoric of foetal rights seems to be largely directed at pregnant women who may wish to end their pregnancy, and the period during which abortion may be sought by the woman herself is limited in the

UK. However, medical decisions to end pregnancy may be made at any time up to the moment of birth if doctors consider the foetus to be severely handicapped (Morris, 1991).

THE RHETORIC OF HELPING

Contentious and even sadistic human actions can be transmuted by nursing language into beneficial interventions. Psychiatric nurses, for example, have long had to be persuaded into a view that interventions they might at first consider to be offensive are in fact therapeutic. Electric shock treatment is an obvious example of this. The softening of what might be thought of as cruel interventions is done through a filter of therapeutic jargon which effectively covers over or erases any

Key reference

initial qualms or reservations about their ethical status. Edelman (1974) writes: 'Because the helping professions define other people's statuses (and their own), the special terms they employ to categorize clients and justify restrictions of their physical movements and of their moral and intellectual influence are especially revealing of the political functions language performs and of the multiple realities it helps create' (p. 296). This is especially the case with the term 'therapy', which converts everyday activities into professional interventions: 'In the journals, textbooks and talk of the helping professions the term is repeatedly used as a suffix or qualifier. Mental patients do not hold dances; they have Dance Therapy. If they play volleyball, that is Recreation Therapy. If they engage in a group discussion, that is Group Therapy. Even reading is "Bibliotherapy" ' (p. 297). This professional appropriation of the everyday, Edelman argues, is a certain means of establishing 'who gives orders and who takes them, and to justify in advance the inhibitions placed upon the subordinate class' (p. 297).

Thus linguistic strategy can enable professionals to believe that they are helping and not repressing those under their care. The language of helping may distort the true picture as in the following example of the difference between an everyday and a professional description of psychiatric interventions:

> A) . . . deprivation of food, bed, walks in the open air, visitors, mail, or telephone calls; solitary confinement; deprivation of reading or entertainment materials; immobilising people by tying them into wet sheets and then exhibiting them to staff and other patients; other physical restraints on body movement; drugging the mind against the client's will; incarceration in locked wards; a range of public humiliations such as the prominent posting of alleged intentions to escape or commit suicide, the requirement of public confessions of misconduct or guilt, and public announcement of individual misdeeds and abnormalities.
>
> (Edelman, 1974, p. 300)

> B) . . . discouraging sick behaviour and encouraging healthy behaviour through the selective granting of rewards; the availability of seclusion, restraints, and closed wards to grant a patient a

respite from interaction with others and from making decisions, and prevent harm to himself or others; enabling him to think about his behaviour, to cope with his temptations to elope and succumb to depression, and to develop a sense of security; immobilising the patient to calm him, satisfy his dependency needs, give him the extra nursing attention he values, and enable him to benefit from peer confrontation; placing limits on his acting out; and teaching him that the staff cares.

(Edelman, 1974, p. 302)

Labelled or diagnosed, the mental patient becomes easy prey for further 'linguistic incarceration' (Crawford, Nolan and Brown, 1995) in what Edelman sees as a tendency to 'seek out data and interpret developments so as to confirm the label and ignore, discount, or reinterpret counter evidence' (p. 300). The language of therapy may override language that depicts what is actually happening. Furthermore, the adoption by clients of the approved linguistic forms relating to their treatment is often seen by staff as evidence of insight and improvement (Edelman, 1974). Disturbingly, Edelman observes that 'The helping professions are the most effective contemporary agents of social conformity and isolation. In playing this political role they engird the entire political structure, yet are largely spared from self-criticism, from political criticism, and even from political observation through a special symbolic language' (p. 310).

Key reference

With wide public support for control of possibly dangerous individuals, the power base of the helping professions looks unlikely to wane. Edelman alerts us to the rhetorical status of nursing language. It can offer particular narrations of care which may well be at odds with reality. The potential for damaging others through language, then, extends beyond notions of how verbal or written mistakes, for example in doses of medicine, can bring serious clinical and professional consequences. The problem of harmful language is much wider and more deeply rooted than this. Perhaps the reason why detrimental aspects of nursing language have largely escaped notice is because of the common-sense view that nursing can only be about helping and healing. Nursing language has too often been thought of as transparent and uncomplicated. But nursing's written and spoken language and its reception of written and spoken communication are inherently value laden and political. Nursing language is where nursing measurement of fellow human beings truly begins. Nurses must remain vigilant to how they are measuring those entrusted to their care in any communication. Only then may nurses be better placed to question how other professions, groups and individuals are measuring them.

CONCLUSIONS

In this chapter we have ranged over a variety of issues relating to language which are important to nursing. We have tried to show how language is central to how we make sense of our world, either as health care professionals or as sufferers from illness, disease or disability. An important conclusion of this argument is to realize that if words are so active, we can do a great deal to modify the experience of care giving or illness by means of the way we talk and write and indeed respond to the talk and writing of others. Clearly, we cannot claim to be able to perform miracle cures, but the realization that we have the freedom to give and receive information provides a much needed sense of control for nurses. If language can cover up or reframe abuses, then it can also expose them. If we realize that we mutually construct versions of our world through language, then sometimes we might want to opt out and refuse to be enlisted. It is sometimes objected that seeing the world in terms of linguistic construction involves us in a murky moral relativism – we can no longer see the difference between truth and falsehood or right and wrong. However, our position can lead to more sensitive ethics in that we can begin to see the strategies people use to make their course of action seem the best or the most ethical. And language is, after all, the arena where they do this.

SUMMARY

In this chapter we have described how language is seldom neutral; it is usually an active force in the social world. The ways in which scholars have attempted to make sense of this, for example by seeing language as a bearer of ideology or as reflecting the multiple, unresolvable stories so beloved of postmodernists, have been described. This enables us to see how important it is to pay attention to language in nursing, as the discipline is centrally concerned with talk, writing, listening and reading. We will devote more attention to listening and reading in chapter 5, on audience. It is also important to be aware of patients' narratives of illness, for it is through these storied processes of sense making that we come to experience illness, whether as a burns victim, a lupus patient or a person undergoing therapy after a head injury. These are all experiences that are narrated and formed into a story that enables them to make sense to the sufferer and any health professionals they encounter. Language is important in all disciplines of nursing, not just the traditionally talk-based ones like psychiatry. How we see patients can systematically influence the kinds of questions that get asked and the types of treatments they receive. Whether we ask a young woman with abdominal pains about contraceptive practices, for example, may well depend on what ethnic group she happens to belong to. Language is important also from the point of view of telling the story of helping. Medical or psychiatric treatments may appear painful or humiliating – it is through language that they are reframed as something beneficial. We have ended with a plea for nurses to be vigilant about how language is used to construct truths or portray the world in a favourable light. It is only by being aware in this way that nurses can safeguard their patients' interests and those of their profession.

REFERENCES

Austin, J.L. (1962) *How to Do Things with Words*, Clarendon Press, Oxford.

Billig, M. (1982) *Ideology and Social Psychology: Extremism, Moderation and Contradiction*, Basil Blackwell, Oxford.

Billig, M., Condor, S., Edwards, D. *et al.* (1987) *Ideological Dilemmas: A Social Psychology of Everyday Thinking*, Sage, London.

Bruner, E.M. (1984) The opening up of anthropology, in *Text, Play and Story: The Construction and Reconstruction of Self and Society* (ed. E.M. Bruner), American Ethnological Society, Washington.

Burke, K. (1945) *A Grammar of Motives*, Prentice Hall, New York.

Charnaz, K. (1991) *Good Days, Bad Days: The Self in Chronic Illness and Time*, Rutgers University Press, New Brunswick, NJ.

Charnaz, K. (1995) Grounded theory, in *Rethinking Methods in Psychology* (eds J. Smith, R. Harre and L. Van Langenhove), Sage, London.

Cheek, J. and Rudge, T. (1994) Nursing as textually mediated reality. *Nursing Inquiry*, 1, 15–22.

Clarke, L. (1996) The last post? Defending nursing against the postmodernist maze. *Journal of Advanced Nursing*, 3, 257–65.

Dale, R. (1976) *Schooling and Capitalism*, Routledge & Kegan Paul, London.

Denzin, N.K. (1989) *Interpretive Biography*, Qualitative Methods Series, 17, Sage, London.

Derrida, J. (1976) *Of Grammatology* (trans. G.C. Spivak), Johns Hopkins University Press, Baltimore.

Dreuilhe, E. (1988) *Mortal Embrace*, Hill & Wang, New York.

Frank, A. (1993) The rhetoric of self change: illness experience as narrative. *Sociological Quarterly*, 34(1), 39–52.

Frazer, E. (1987) Teenage girls reading *Jackie*. *Media, Culture and Society*, 9, 407–25.

Garvin, B.J., Kennedy, C.W., Baker, C.F., and Polivka, B.J. (1992) Cardiovascular responses of CCU patients when communicating with nurses, physicians, and families. *Health Communication*, 4(4), 291–301.

Ginsburg, N. (1980) *Class, Capital and Social Policy*, Macmillan, London.

Good, B. (1990) *The Narrative Representation of Illness*, Lewis Henry Morgan Lectures, University of Rochester, Rochester, NY.

Graumann, C.F. (1984) Unbalancing social psychology. *Contemporary Psychology*, 29, 281–3.

Grice, H.P. (1975) Logic and conversation, in *Syntax and Semantics 3: Speech Acts* (eds P. Cole and J.P. Morgan), Academic Press, New York.

Griffin, C. (1992) Fear of a black (and working class) planet: young women and the radicalisation of reproductive politics. *Feminism and Psychology*, 2, 491–4.

Hays, J.C. (1989) Voices in the record. *IMAGE: Journal of Nursing Scholarship*, 21(4), 200–4.

Henriques, J., Hollway, W., Venn, C. and Walkerdine, V. (1984) *Changing the Subject: Psychology, Social Regulation and Subjectivity*, Methuen, London.

Herzlich, C. and Pierret, J. (1987) *Illness and Self in Society*, Johns Hopkins University Press, Baltimore

Hunt, A., Litt, I. and Loebner, M. (1988) Obtaining a sexual history from adolescent girls: a preliminary report of the influence of age and ethnicity. *Journal of Adolescent Health Care*, 9, 52–4.

Hyden, M. (1992) Woman battering as marital act: the construction of a violent marriage. Doctoral dissertation, University of Stockholm, Stockholm.

Jensen, K.B. (1987) Qualitative audience research: towards an integrative approach to reception. *Critical Studies in Mass Communication*, 4, 21–36.

Kleinman, A. (1988) *The Illness Narratives: Suffering, Healing and the Human Condition*, Basic Books, New York.

Language acts

Labov, W. (1972) The transformation of experience in narrative syntax, in *Language in the Inner City: Studies in the Black English Vernacular* (ed. W. Labov), University of Pennsylvania Press, Philadelphia.

Labov, W. (1982) Speech actions and reactions in personal narrative, in *Georgetown Round Table in Languages and Linguistics* (ed. D. Tannen), Georgetown University Press, Washington.

Labov, W. and Waletzky, J. (1967) Narrative analysis: oral versions of personal experience, in *Essays on the Verbal and Visual Arts* (ed. J. Helm), University of Washington Press, Seattle.

Lempert, L.B. (1994) A narrative analysis of abuse: connecting the personal, the rhetorical and the structural. *Journal of Contemporary Ethnography*, 22(4), 411–41.

Leonard, P. (1984) *Personality and Ideology: Towards a Materialist Understanding of the Individual*, Macmillan, London.

Levine, M.E. (1989) The ethics of nursing rhetoric. *Image: Journal of Nursing Scholarship*, 21(1), 4–6.

Manzo, J.F., Blonder, L.X. and Burns, A.F. (1995) The social-interactional organisation of narrative and narrating among stroke patients and their spouses. *Sociology of Health and Illness*, 17(3), 307–27.

Mattingly, C. (1994) The concept of therapeutic emplotment. *Social Science and Medicine*, 38(6), 811–22.

May, W.F. (1991) *The Patient's Ordeal*, Indiana University Press, Bloomington.

Morris, J. (1991) *Pride against Prejudice: Transforming Attitudes to Disability*, Women's Press, London.

Parry, N., Rustin, M. and Satyamurti, C. (1979) (eds) *Social Work, Welfare and the State*, Edward Arnold, London.

Ricouer, P. (1991) Life quest of narrative, in *On Paul Ricouer: Narrative and Interpretation* (ed. D. Wood) Routledge, London.

Rosenwald, G.C. and Ochberg, R.L. (1992) *Storied Lives: The Cultural Politics of Self Understanding*, Yale University Press, New Haven.

Scannell, P., Schlesinger, P. and Sparks, C. (1992) (eds) *Culture and Power: A Media, Culture and Society Reader*, Sage, London.

Searle, J. (1969) *Speech Acts: An Essay in the Philosophy of Language*, Cambridge University Press, London.

Stedman-Jones, G. (1971) *Outcast London*, Clarendon Press, Oxford.

Therborn, G. (1980) *The Ideology of Power and the Power of Ideology*, Verso, London.

Thomas, S.A., Friedmann, E., Lottes, L.S. *et al.* (1984) Changes in nurses' blood pressure and heart rate while communicating. *Research in Nursing and Health*, 7, 119–26.

UKCC (1993) *Standards for Records and Record Keeping*, United Kingdom Central Council for Nursing Midwifery and Health Visiting, London.

Walker, K. (1995) Nursing, narrativity and research: towards a poetics and politics of orality. *Contemporary Nurse*, 4(4), 156–63.

Wilson, E. (1977) *Women and the Welfare State*, Tavistock, London.

Yoshida, K.K. (1993) Reshaping the self: a pendular reconstruction of self and identity among adults with traumatic spinal cord injury. *Sociology of Health and Illness*, 15(2), 217–45.

KEY REFERENCES

Bertens, H. (1995) *The Idea of the Postmodern: A History*, Routledge, London.

Bolinger, D. (1980) *Language: The Loaded Weapon*, Longman, London.

Crawford, P., Nolan, P. and Brown, B. (1995) Linguistic entrapment: medico-nursing biographies as fictions. *Journal of Advanced Nursing*, 22, 1141–8.

Edelman, M. (1974) The political language of the helping professions. *Politics and Society*, 4, 295–310.

Fairclough, N. (1989) *Language and Power*, Longman, London.

Mathieson, C.M. and Stam, H.J. (1995) Re-negotiating identity: cancer narratives. *Sociology of Health and Illness*, 17(3), 283–306.

Riessman, C.K. (1993) *Narrative Analysis*, Qualitative Research Methods Series, 30, Sage, London.

2 AUTHORSHIP: WHO TELLS?

AIMS

This chapter aims to show how nurses are not the sole authors of either spoken or written texts, since what they say and write is constructed from texts that originate elsewhere, not least texts introduced during their professional training and subsequent socialization as practising nurses.

In particular, this chapter aims to challenge the view that what nurses say or write simply reflects the state of the world. Nurse authorship is strongly influenced by cultural, legal, organizational and political contexts. A variety of constraints act upon nursing language. We will discuss the importance of the narration of illness to nursing records. We will show that nursing narratives of patients' illnesses can never be impartial. Finally, this chapter points out the limited storytelling rights of nurses and suggests that they need to consider new ways of enhancing their status as authors.

INTRODUCTION: THE CONTEXT OF AUTHORSHIP

In this chapter, the issue of authorship in nursing practice is examined. The sheer pervasiveness of language in health care makes this an important issue. Whether as clients or nursing professionals, researchers, administrators or policy makers, our actions through language constitute a vital part of the health care system. Whatever our role, we are all authors speaking or writing the language of health care. Barker (1996, p. 242) notes that 'care for the person *as a whole*' is problematic, especially 'given that the whole person can only be understood linguistically (Stevenson, 1996)', so that in the discipline of psychiatry 'nursing is predicated upon mutual authoring and re-authoring (Hulme, 1996)'. Whatever their discipline, all nurses need to gain a greater awareness of their position as authors of health care. In order to progress to an understanding of how nurses may actively participate in re-authoring or reshaping health care stories, it is necessary to examine further the complex issues surrounding authorship itself.

The complex social functions of language can be difficult to grasp because we tend to think of language as transparent. In Europe and North America, we grow up with the idea that we are the sole authors of what we say, write and do. One of the first questions that springs to mind when we see a piece of writing is to ask who wrote it. The idea is that the writing reflects the values, personality and attitudes of the writer. Speech and writing are assumed to tell us what that individual is thinking or doing.

Recent scholarship in linguistics, cultural studies and discourse analysis suggests that there is a great deal more to it than this.

Example 1

Communication is enabled through the use of standard forms of words, ideas, images and phrases which originated elsewhere and which we pick up as we learn the language or train as health care professionals.

A further unspoken assumption in European and North American cultures is that language reflects the state of the world – words are names for things; sentences describe nature and may do so truthfully or falsely. 'The cat sat on the mat' or 'The quick brown fox jumps over the lazy dog', for example, describe the relationship between objects in the world with more or less accuracy. However, many scholars (Edwards and Potter, 1992; Psathas, 1995) argue that the most important aspect of language is how it is used to perform items of social business. Language is how we get things done. To understand language in nursing is to understand the functions it performs. These functions are not simple, but are every bit as complex as whatever we can imagine is going on between a large number of people in an organizational setting such as a hospital or community care team. Language cannot be separated from the complex human activity that gives it shape and meaning.

Certainly, language is spoken and written by individuals but the things they say in health care are influenced by many things. A preliminary list might include:

(1) The values, norms and attitudes that we draw upon from the wider cultural context.
(2) The specific terms and concepts that we learn through being trained in health care; the historical controversies that have resulted in their being understood as they are today.
(3) The legal and organizational context – what our superiors want and what the law requires.
(4) The common-sense means of interpreting what patients tell staff and staff tell each other.
(5) The organization's policies relating to record keeping; the forms, rating scales, standard diagnostic interviews which staff are supposed to use.
(6) The broader political context which dictates acceptable terminology in health care, appropriate treatments, and the time allocated to patients.

EXAMPLE 1: LANGUAGE MEANS MONEY, LANGUAGE CHANGES

Most people will agree that using appropriate terms to describe a patient's condition is one aspect of professionalism, but in recent times the economics and politics of health care have infiltrated more strongly the language used by carers and clients. At the time of writing, the US nursing press is concerned with the issue of current procedural terminology (CPT) in nursing practice. As well as being a standardized way of describing nursing, CPT is vitally important in the claiming of payment for services (Griffith and Robinson, 1993). The message is clear – the language nurses use makes all the difference between financial success or failure. A quick glance at history reveals many more examples of the same thing; for example, nineteenth-century philanthropists were successful in raising funds to help 'fallen women'. It is unlikely that these stalwarts of Victorian morality would have been so successful had they asked for money to help prostitutes or whores. Economic constraints on the language used in health care contexts mean that descriptions of human distress and disease are, in an important sense, expressions of our culture.

The terms and concepts available to characterize what is wrong with people have shifted dramatically in the last 150 years. The popularity that the diagnosis of 'masturbatory insanity' enjoyed in the nineteenth century waned as the twentieth century wore on. Kraepelin's 'dementia praecox' was replaced by Bleuler's 'schizophrenia'. Gull's work on 'anorexia nervosa' or 'nervous loss of appetite' in 1874 ushered in an era of medical concern with young women's size, shape and eating patterns.

EXAMPLE 2: LANGUAGE REFLECTS POLITICS

The last 20 years have furnished whole new vocabularies for describing human distress and disease. In 1981, the prestigious *New England Journal of Medicine* carried a paper by Gottleib describing an unusual pattern of pneumonia and candida infection in gay men. The authors coined the term 'GRID' (gay related immune deficiency) for what they had observed, as the only characteristic that appeared to link these men was that they were practising homosexuals. As the condition was detected in other groups of people, GRID was changed to 'AIDS' (acquired immune deficiency syndrome). Many educators, activists and gay men were concerned not to identify AIDS too closely in the public mind with homosexuality for fear of fuelling homophobia and anti-gay violence and encouraging a rapid spread of HIV infection among heterosexuals who presumed they were not at risk (Gorna, 1996). Thus the UK's public health message promoted the idea that 'AIDS is everyone's issue' and 'HIV is an equal opportunities virus'. Popular UK publications carried articles such as 'Meet a girl like you who's HIV positive' (*Cosmopolitan*, January 1991, quoted in Gorna, 1996, p. 11). The AIDS scare shows how names for diseases and thinking about them are crucially informed by the politics, values and prejudices of contemporary society.

EXAMPLE 3: WHAT DOES A DIAGNOSTIC CATEGORY MEAN? UNPACKING THE MYSTERY OF EATING DISORDERS

A third example of how the stories health carers tell about human distress are part of historical and linguistic culture is provided by the contentious area of eating disorders. Since the time when Gull coined

Example 3

the term 'anorexia nervosa' and Lasegue identified 'anorexie hysterique' in 1874, anorexia has attracted much scholarship and debate. The other major category of eating disorder, bulimia nervosa, which involves bingeing and purging, was identified more recently and placed on the research agenda only by Russell's paper in 1979. Yet estimates of its prevalence suggest that in the early 1990s, 1–6 per cent of young women were affected (American Psychiatric Association, 1994; Rand and Kuldau, 1992; Bennet, Spoth and Borgen, 1991). So what Russell saw as an ominous variant of anorexia nervosa is now listed in most textbooks and in the influential *Diagnostic and Statistical Manual* (DSM) of the American Psychiatric Association (1994) as a disorder in its own right.

Today, different communities of people talk about the problems of anorexia and bulimia nervosa in different ways. The very term 'eating disorder' is contentious. Many feminist authors, such as Burstow (1992), object to it, arguing that the eating habits of people who are diagnosed in this way are anything but disordered. Rather, they are meticulously organized. It is only the clinicians and researchers who identify them as disordered. Thus, Burstow prefers the term 'troubled eating'. The language used is crucial to the way in which the debate is conducted. Many critics of psychiatry consider diagnostic categories to be laden with political and sexual stereotyping which should be challenged. 'Troubled eating' is argued to be a better term because it indicates more clearly the sufferer's personal distress and the distress of those close to her without incorporating the negative and stigmatizing implications associated with a mental disorder label.

Understanding language is crucial to understanding why the apparently simple matter of saying that someone has anorexia nervosa is really not so simple. Researchers, clinicians and professional bodies have tried to identify criteria that characterize eating disorders. The major diagnostic schemes in common use, the US DSM and the International Classification of Diseases (or ICD; World Health Organisation, 1992), try to define criteria according to the distilled wisdom of the research literature and the practice of member states. This type of corporate authorship is common in psychiatry. To diagnose someone as having an eating disorder is to apply the criteria from the learned tomes which describe the criteria originated by committees, conferences and experts. Our thinking and speech about eating disorders reproduce language – authorship – that lies elsewhere. When we use the terms devised by prestigious corporate authors, we are participating in a broader set of social relations.

Diagnostic categories conceal ambiguity, debate and disagreement. The DSM and ICD do not agree on a definition of anorexia. The DSM says that in order to have a diagnosis of anorexia nervosa, a sufferer must be at 85 per cent or less of the appropriate weight for her or his age and height. The ICD, on the other hand, does not specify a particular weight limit, and a further influential set of criteria devised by Dally *et al.* (1979) suggest that sufferers' weight must be more than 10 per cent below normal. Although there is broad agreement about the presentation of eating disorders, there are nevertheless significant differences in how the respected texts in the field define them.

These inconsistencies are only the beginning. The diagnostic criteria gloss over a vigorous debate as to where the line should be drawn between ordinary and disordered eating. In *The Diagnosis and Treatment of Normal Eating* Polivy and Herman (1987) argue that for many women in the USA ordinary eating and concerns about their weight and shape have features in common with eating disorders. Attempts have been made to define eating disorders in such a way as to separate them from whatever normal eating might be. For example, Crisp (1980) is at pains to draw a distinction between anorexia and ordinary dieting. Anorexics, he argues, pursue thinness for different reasons than dieters. Dieters want to lose weight, whereas anorexic adolescents are undergoing a maturational crisis and are unable to meet the psychosocial demands of puberty. Crisp (1980) presents a series of accounts from anorexic women to illustrate why, in his view, anorexia is a set of bizarre and abnormal experiences. However, Chesters (1994) had no difficulty in finding a number of young women who had never been diagnosed as anorexic but who said very similar things to Crisp's patients. Compare the following:

From Crisp (1980, pp. 158–9):

> 'I was terrified of gaining weight.'

From Chesters (1994, p. 453):

> Interviewer: 'How would you feel if you gained ten pounds?'
> S10: 'Very panicked, very panicked, ummm like because I step on the scales every day or if not every day at least three times a week, it wouldn't, I wouldn't just do it because at the moment if I get to eight and a half stone a light sort of red light would begin to come on, if I had put on 10 pounds I would feel panicked, I would go into dieting mode.'

As Chesters comments, this subject speaks in a very similar way to Crisp's patient and uses emergency terminology such as red lights going on. Thus it is difficult to tell the difference between patient and non-patient. It is difficult to sustain the argument that disorders are simply or unproblematically there in the patients. The professional framework that is brought to bear on patients' behaviour, speech and thinking is used to make sense of what is going on.

What has been said about the limitations of a diagnosis of anorexia could equally well be applied to other disorders such as schizophrenia, a concept powerfully criticized by Mary Boyle (1990, 1992, 1994), or paranoia which David Harper (1992, 1994, 1996) has shown is a diagnosis serving the interests of professionals and professional ideologies rather than simply being a description of patients' thoughts.

The story we tell about clients' distress is, therefore, crucially informed by the frames of reference that we have available to us. Moreover, it often turns out that these ways of making clinical sense are formulated differently by different authors. Language thus performs an important function in glossing over the cracks in nature and the cracks in professional practice. If, in fact, we had no way of performing this glossing-over function, caring would be a very difficult business indeed. The complex nature of many people's problems would mean health professionals would have to start from scratch every time they met a client, whereas the pre-authored categories and diagnoses mean that all that is needed is to adapt what is seen and heard to fit the authorship that others have already performed.

TELLING STORIES ABOUT DISTRESS: FROM MODERNISM TO POSTMODERNISM

Health professionals make sense of the world in which they work by drawing on the resources of meaning with which their culture and training provide them. This is not surprising, as the scientific story we learn about the practice of health care has a sense of coherence and optimism. Since the eighteenth century, sometimes known as the Age of Reason, the belief that the world will yield its secrets to scientific inquiry has been extremely popular in Europe and the United States (Hollinger, 1994). This belief is associated with the view that rational, systematic means of acquiring knowledge are the best, and that knowledge should be based on scientifically derived facts.

The distinction between modernism and postmodernism can be seen at work here. Modernism is the perspective still taken by most textbooks of psychology, psychiatry and nursing, which carefully avoid what the authors consider to be myths, superstitions or metaphysics. Modernism is associated with what has been called an 'up the mountain' theory of science which proclaims that we know far more now than we ever did in the past, and that practice and treatment are getting better as time goes on. The *naïveté* and cruelty of medicine and nursing in the past are contrasted with the enlightened, humane and caring approach of the present day. The modernist point of view (e.g. Ritzer, 1992) is often sustained by some grand narrative as to the nature of the material world, such as the idea that human consciousness can ultimately be explained in terms of brain chemistry. Michel Foucault has argued that, from its inception, 'The science of man . . . was medically based' (1975, p. 36). The education of health professionals is pervaded with such assumptions.

Allied to this outlook is the notion that individuals are the authors of their own ideas, speech or writing. From Descartes' assertion 'I think; therefore, I am', to contemporary concern with individuals' thoughts, emotions and actions, the idea of authorship or responsibility has been essential to the sciences and humanities.

Postmodernism takes a very different stance. Postmodernists do not find the world to be ordered and coherent and consider grand narratives doomed to failure. Postmodernism is a loose collection of philosophies that emphasize difference rather than unity, fragmentation rather than integration, and the minority or unusual point of view rather than the majority or mainstream viewpoint. As we noted in chapter 1, postmodern thinkers are often concerned with language: 'Language is now necessarily the central consideration in all attempts to know, act and live' (Lemert, 1990, p. 234). Lyotard (1984), Lemert (1990) and Ritzer (1992) all view scientific theories as texts – we usually encounter them in written form. Furthermore, the empirical reality to which scientific theories apply is often textual. In nursing, care plans, patient records and the wider body of theory and research on which practice is based are all texts. Almost every part of health care, certainly as it is performed by people directly involved with clients, is mediated through language. Clarke (1996) argues that a postmodernist perspective requires nurses to 'connect with the devolved needs/wants of patients, in respect of their autonomy and medication, and cease pursuing abstract, doctrinaire ideals' (p. 261).

Postmodernism encourages a greater sensitivity to the local concerns of patients. For many years, nursing education was a matter of learning about hygiene, practising techniques and memorizing procedures: the grand narratives of biomedical models of health. More recently, nursing thinking has come to emphasize more strongly the caring role of nurses and the importance of nurses reflecting critically on their practice. This might be described as the beginnings of a postmodern consciousness among nurses.

Key reference

The importance of texts in nursing has been increasingly recognized as scholars strive to understand the nursing process. As Cheek and Rudge (1994) say, 'nursing and nursing practice can be considered to represent a reality which is textually mediated' (p. 15). The turn to texts in nursing scholarship is also associated with a scepticism of 'grand narratives' – Darbyshire (1994) warns us away from sets of abstract principles in making sense of nursing practice. The postmodern concern with minority points of view has led some to ask why conventional nursing research ignores the 40 million Americans without health care (Allen, 1995).

The question of 'Who tells?' is a huge one. It encompasses the language produced by health service users themselves, their relatives and friends and the language of nurses, social workers and doctors as well as of a range of other people with whom users come into contact. To begin to unravel the question of 'Who tells?' involves making sense of the historical, professional and academic background of what is said and exploring how health carers deploy the resources of their professional wisdom on the raw material of clients' accounts of their troubles.

MAKING SENSE OF EACH OTHER: COMMON SENSE, INTERPRETIVE COMMUNITIES, GENRES AND REGISTERS

One of the first people to theorize about common sense was the Italian philosopher Antonio Gramsci. During his imprisonment by Mussolini,

Gramsci wrote about common sense as something that includes 'prejudice from all past phases in history at the local level and intuitions of a future philosophy which will be that of the human race united the world over' (Gramsci, 1971, p. 321).

Common sense is not a unified body of knowledge; perhaps it is best seen as a storehouse of knowledge that has been gathered together historically through struggle and dispute. Confrontation between gay and lesbian activists and the American Psychiatric Association in the early 1970s led to the removal of homosexuality from the *Diagnostic and Statistical Manual*. However, many of the more conservative members of the profession retained a lingering belief that homosexuality was unhealthy, as is clear from fairly recent attempts to identify lesbianism as 'a symptom of neurosis and a grievous personality disorder' (Kronemeyer, 1980, p. 14; see also Kitzinger, 1986, p. 151).

Contemporary feminist scholars (e.g. Kitzinger and Perkins, 1993; Kitzinger, 1993) have argued persuasively that heterosexist assumptions are pervasive among carers. As Perkins (1996, p. 17) reports, 'Recent studies of the attitudes of nurses in the UK and USA show that as many as 40 per cent would not condone homosexuality. A minority claim the right not to treat lesbian and gay patients and some even see AIDS as a divine punishment' (Taylor and Robertson, 1994).

Thus we can identify the way in which common sense develops through a process of struggle. Gramsci suggested that common sense embodies the practical solutions to everyday problems and that it does this by 'being richly shot through with elements and beliefs derived from earlier or other more developed ideologies which have sedimented into it' (quoted in Hall *et al*. 1978, p. 154).

The common frames of understanding, what Hawes (1977) called 'situated logics-in-use', are important in understanding postmodernism. Most postmodernist philosophies are anti-foundationalist – that is, they do not propose that our knowledge rests on a single version of reason (Hollinger, 1994). Rather they consider that truth is established interpersonally and that systems of logic or ideas about the world are often parochial and local (Geertz, 1983). The climate of problematization fostered by postmodernism has encouraged scholars to examine how patients, therapists, nurses and psychiatrists structure illness problems.

The vocabulary of health care concepts and care plans in nursing does not simply reflect patients and their problems. These problems are not simply told by the professional whose handwriting appears in the patients' records. Language looks as it does because of its history in science, institutional care and education, and its contemporary social functions. Over time, a community of understanding is established in which technical terms such as 'agoraphobia' or 'schizophrenia' have a common meaning, and where non-technical terms such as 'progress' are managed so that the evolution in patients' behaviour is formulated to ensure that therapy appears to be effective.

Given that members of the health professions spend so much time talking to, writing about and interacting with clients, it is startling that they do not already have some theory of health care communication. However, insight can be gained by looking to the disciplines of literature and communication studies. Fish (1980) proposed the idea of an interpretive community, a group of writers and readers who share assumptions about the production and reading of texts and what they mean. The health professions might be seen as such an interpretive community.

There are a great many formal processes in the life of health professionals, such as education, training and professional development, which generate this common frame of understanding. Radway (1984) examined some of these processes at work in a community of readers of romantic novels. The members of the community shared a common purpose in that all were housewives; as a result of their reading and interaction with each other, the women developed a group preference, favouring stories that described a stormy relationship between one man and one woman which culminated in marriage. How does this apply to nursing? Radway's study suggests that other groups, such as nurses, work together to fix meaning and to communicate it to others. Lindlof (1988) tried to define more exactly what an interpretive community is. From his point of view, our language and interaction do not simply reflect a reality that is out there, but are constructed by the community. The kind of language and understanding generated by the community is distinctive. For example, at a Midlands hospital that has suffered from occasional outbreaks of MRSA – a soft tissue infection that attacks open wounds and is especially difficult to eradicate – a familiar quip among nurses is that 'Mrs A's on the ward again.' The infection is described like a familiar patient. Although the medical features of MRSA are still being scrutinized, nurses use this jocular expression to cut the additional work and distress caused by the infection down to size. The term 'Mrs A' is particular to this nursing community.

Nurses' talk and writing about the way they deliver care is directed to a particular audience. The narratives of schizophrenia in the psychiatric literature, for example, differ radically from those used to educate anxious parents about why their previously promising son is neglecting his studies and complaining that he is hearing voices. These accounts of care look very different according to whether they are intended to stay within one community or to cross boundaries between communities.

The notion of a community of understanding has much in common with the idea of genre in literary studies, where the language used in particular contexts is characterized by certain regularities (Bhatia, 1993; Swales, 1990; Ventola, 1988; Martin, 1984). A wide variety of genres or 'conventions which arise from preferred ways of creating and communicating knowledge within particular communities' (Swales, 1990, p. 4) operate in health care. For example, medical staff involved in organ transplantation look for organs to 'harvest', as in the case of eye specialists seeking material for corneal grafts, who might visit the intensive care unit and ask jovially, 'Got any eyes?'

Nurses might be uncomfortable with such language because it goes against the grain of the caring atmosphere they are trying to create. This is just one example of the many ways in which care staff can participate in different genres of speech and writing, each of which is felt to be suitable within a specific context.

Proctor, Morse and Khonsari's study (1996) of how nurses in a trauma centre in a US hospital talk to injured patients uses some of these concepts of genre. By videotaping interactions between nurses and patients in pain, the authors identified what they called the 'comfort talk register'. The register was rather like a genre in that it involved different kinds of talk with specific pragmatic functions. The researchers identified four functions: holding on, assessing, informing, and caring.

Key reference

(1) *Holding on* was conducted through the use of phrases like 'big girl', 'you're doing great', 'count to three'. This served to praise, to let the patient know they can get through, to support, to instruct or distract the patient.
(2) *Assessing* involved 'How are you?' questions or giving the patient information – 'you're in the emergency room'. These concerned obtaining information, explaining the situation or validating and confirming the patient's input.
(3) *Informing* involved statements like 'it's gonna hurt' or 'we'll be inserting a catheter'. These involved warning the patient or explaining procedures.
(4) *Caring* included statements like 'relax' or 'OK sweetie' or 'it does hurt, doesn't it?' – in other words some sort of reassurance, empathy or caring comment (p. 1673).

The authors suggest that because these features of comfort talk are regularly used, the talk has a rhythmical quality and is mainly used to get patients to endure the situation a little longer. The comfort talk register was delivered with greater than normal volume, in short, simple sentences, and using a restricted range of linguistic devices to give it a singsong quality. The study concludes that the comfort talk probably helped to reduce the morbidity and mortality of trauma patients.

This particular piece of research highlights what can be detected when language in health settings is taken as a topic of enquiry in its own right, and relations between form and function are explored.

SPEAKING OTHER PEOPLE'S LINES

Whereas the study of genre and register is characterized by interest in the *form* of communicative acts, it is also important to attend to the conventions and patterns of content and meaning. Many items in the present-day vocabulary of nursing originated in the nineteenth or early twentieth century. In a sense, nurses are speaking other people's lines.

Goffman (1981) used the idea of *footing* to describe the way in which speakers signal that they are reporting the speech of others. He contrasts the *animator* who is doing the talking and the *composer* who originally made up the words. Footing is one of the ways in which speakers display the accountability of what they say. In nursing, this may be explicit as when people quote from some textbook, manual, paper or scientific study, authoritative source or set of guidelines to add credentials to a course of action. However, simply using a technical term or specialized vocabulary without citing the source can signal that the speaker is familiar with the work of the (often prestigious) composers of the terminology and thus should be considered to be saying something fundamentally rational.

Edwards and Potter (1992) identify problems with the concept of footing because a great deal of the talk in everyday contexts is made up of widely held views, ideas and commonplaces and employs conventional rhetorical devices for telling factual accounts (see Billig, 1989a, 1989b; Moscovici, 1984; Wooffitt, 1992) where it is not clear who the composers and originators of the language were. The work of Lacan (1977) and Foucault (1965) shifts the focus from authors and originators to texts, discourses and frames of understanding that are wider than individuals. The various talk and writing of psychiatry, for example, may be recirculated and reproduced in the literature but does not necessarily have identifiable originators. What can be detected is a correspondence between the technical literature and what people say or write – so-called intertextuality (Curt, 1994). This involves people using and absorbing and, indeed, even transforming what others have said or written before them.

Shotter's (1993) ideas about social accountability are also relevant in understanding the language of health care. He argues that in order to be socially competent, we must be able to account for our actions as being those of fully autonomous adults. By 'accountable', Shotter does not mean that we continually justify our behaviour but that we're more or less aware of whether our actions match the social rules of rationality. However, at the same time, our accounts are often 'joint transactions' with other people and therefore disorderly (see Shotter, 1993, p. 168). Nursing records embody some of these processes when the messy business of talking with patients is compressed into socially acceptable and technical terms such as 'agoraphobia' (Fairclough, 1989). The complexity of patients' feelings about their problems is formulated into goals and subsequent nursing activity becomes an examination of whether these goals are achieved. The records fit in a justifiable way into the forms of rationality promoted in the education of doctors, nurses and other therapists and fit in with the institutional practices of the hospital.

We cannot therefore assume that the narratives that find their way into the literature of nursing are a transparent rendering of what is going on inside clients' heads. The narratives might be affected by factors such as the genres in which the narratives are produced.

It is not difficult to find examples of texts that provide explicit instructions as to how professionals can give the right kind of accounts of patients in their care. The *Concise Oxford Textbook of Psychiatry*

(Gelder, Gath and Mayou, 1994) defines what makes a good description of a patient: 'Relevant features should be summarized in a few phrases that would give a clear picture to someone who has not met the patient. For example: 'a tall, gaunt, stooping, and dishevelled man with a sad countenance who looks much older than his 40 years' (p. 29).

It is extraordinary that such an account is presented as good practice. We can see here how student health care professionals are encouraged into value-laden and pejorative descriptions of their clients. Who is to judge what constitutes a *dishevelled* appearance? How should someone of 40 look and in what ways does this man appear to be older? How would being encouraged to make this kind of judgement affect a psychiatrist's perception of someone from a different ethnic group? Or someone from a distinctive subcultural group? Although this quote is directed at trainee psychiatrists, we should be alert to the possibility of it happening in nursing and other health care disciplines too. How exactly are we being encouraged to write about those in our care?

As well as explicit instruction from teachers and textbooks, the training of a health professional involves informal processes of socialization. There are a variety of communication practices that might be objected to by patients or frowned on by the authorities if they were discovered. For instance, professionals develop informal diagnostic criteria and category names for patients. Becker (1993; Becker *et al.* 1961) describes how medical students in Kansas in the 1950s characterized some patients as 'crocks'. In discussions with Becker, the students began by suggesting that crocks had psychosomatic complaints. However, this was eventually decided not to be the meaning as a senior physician had used the term when discussing a patient with an observable physical pathology in the form of an ulcer. Eventually they decided that crocks were patients who had complaints but no observable physical pathology. The process of creating informal diagnoses, then, is by no means obvious, even to people involved in it.

Calling patients 'crocks' is an example of 'back space talk' (Goffman, 1981), for use when patients cannot overhear. Communicating like this may lead to complications if patients do hear, for example in cases where staff have assumed patients to be anaesthetized when they were in fact conscious of what was being said about them (Kiviniemi, 1994). Another example concerns a man who survived tetanus in the 1930s but spent several months, paralysed, in hospital. Much later in his life, he recalled how staff would say to each other: 'He hasn't got long' or 'Innee dead yet?'

So there is not one form of telling or communicating, but several. Informal talk involves terms and concepts that would not find their way into formal records or a formal consultation with a patient. Health pro- fessionals become literate in a variety of styles or genres and are able to deploy them in appropriate or, as can happen, completely inappropriate circumstances.

STORIES OF SICKNESS, STORIES OF COPING AND
STORIES OF MAKING SENSE: THE INTERPLAY BETWEEN
CLIENTS' AND PROFESSIONALS' FRAMES OF AUTHORSHIP

When we consider European or North American white majority
cultures, the degree of correspondence between the stories told by
patients and professionals makes it easy to take the signs, symptoms,
syndromes and illnesses for granted. However, it is important to
realize that if we shift the cultural frame of reference a little, the
problems people express may seem to be at odds with dominant
western medical notions of health and illness. Sachs's (1983) account
of Turkish women resident in Sweden illustrates this point:

> In the forty days after childbirth known as the *lohusa* period, a
> woman is liable to contract *albasmasi*. This condition, charac-
> terised by the woman seeing everything in red, turning hot and
> getting cramps as well as choking, is one of the most feared
> reactions connected with childbirth. All women have heard of it
> and been in touch with it one way or another in Kulu. *Albasmasi*
> is an illness with specific symptoms. When a case has been
> established, it is only the personal and folk sectors of health care
> that can provide treatment. A scientific doctor will not be con-
> sulted. The Kulu women know that only their own experts can
> cure a person from *albasmasi* and that scientific doctors have not
> even heard of the illness. (p. 86)

In this case, debate might revolve around the extent to which
albasmasi is similar to postnatal depression, and whether the treatment might be akin to the placebo effect or Euro-American concepts
of psychotherapy. Carr and Vitaliano (1985) ask whether disorders
are particular to specific cultures or 'simply culturally determined
variants of universal forms of psychopathology like depression?'
(p. 244).

The extent to which we can see similarities between illnesses in
different contexts depends in part on how we structure the problem.
The approach in most large-scale cross-cultural studies is the standardized questionnaire or interview format such as the Present State
examination used in the International Pilot Study of Schizophrenia
(Sartorius, Shapiro and Jablonsky, 1974). Some authors (Kleinman,
1987; Bracken, 1993) argue that the supposed similarity in schizophrenia in different nations is merely a result of using this standard
instrument and that many of the most interesting questions about
how the experiences of the interviewees are made sense of in their
particular culture are ignored.

One of the informants in Fenton and Sadiq-Sangster's (1996)
study commented, 'My heart is weak. I am ill with too much thinking
. . . the blood becomes weaker with worry . . . I have the illness of
sorrows' (p. 75). This was a woman of South Asian parentage
speaking after her nephew had died in an accident. Can this account
be repackaged by the interviewer as 'depression', or does labelling

what she is suffering as 'depression' lose some of the culturally important information which could lead to her being helped?

To make connections between stories of distress told by clients and dominant European or American ideas, the researchers in this study had to work quite hard to make sense of one in terms of the other. The terms in which nurses are told about people's troubles do not necessarily translate easily into what they have learned from the textbooks. Because much medical research is conducted from a European or American point of view, many researchers tend to see other culture's problems as masked versions of their own (Patel and Winston, 1994). Ndetei and Muhangi (1979) report that anxiety and depression were the commonest problems at a rural clinic in Kenya. Yet they say that 'none of the patients complained of subjective symptoms of either apprehension or fearfulness in the case of anxiety' (p. 270). Likewise, there was a lack of 'sadness, guilt or nihilism in the case of depression' (p. 270). Even 'direct enquiry about these feeling states also failed to elicit positive responses' (p. 270). It would appear that the power of the language of western diagnostic systems enabled even the absence of key features of anxiety and depression to be glossed over or ignored in the eagerness to find a diagnosis.

The story of distress has, therefore, to be filtered and understood through professional frames of understanding. Willis (1980) argues that 'there is no truly untheoretical way in which to 'see' an 'object'. The 'object' is only perceived and understood through an internal organisation of data, mediated by conceptual constructs and ways of seeing the world. The final account of an object says as much about the observer as it does about the object itself' (p. 90).

It is important to note that even scientific terms used to describe mental and physical illnesses have a metaphorical quality (Sontag, 1979), that is, they may be applied to objects to which they are not literally applicable. People's descriptions of symptoms are burdened with other meanings even when they are talking about apparently clear-cut areas such as alcoholism or agoraphobia. Migliore (1993) **Key reference** describes the way Sicilian-Canadians use the idea of 'nerves' to 'express feelings of concern and distress over their social situation. They translate social problems into the metaphorical language of psychic and somatic distress' (p. 343). 'Nerves' operates as an illness category and as a device for metaphorically expressing a variety of personal and social problems.

Metaphors of illness are especially powerful. As Ricouer (1977) puts it, 'Metaphor is the rhetorical process by which discourse unleashes the power that certain fictions have to redescribe reality' (p. 7). Some theorists, such as Lakoff (1987), argue even more radically not only that metaphor influences how we perceive reality but also that it can structure how we experience that reality.

The way people described the experience of health and illness in a Mexican community studied by Castro (1995) was intimately bound up with their social circumstances. To the impoverished inhabitants of Ocuituco, the terms used to describe illness and wellness relate to material circumstances. To be healthy is to be *gordo*, which means fat, fleshy or stout. To be ill is to be *flaco*, which means thin. Health, then, is conceptualized as fat, with the implication that one is having enough to eat.

The metaphorical and socially embedded quality of descriptions of health and disease are important in understanding the accounts of distress from other cultures. In the case of 'nerves' or attitudes towards food, this can be an easy case to make. However, it is important to bear in mind that similar considerations can illuminate the experience of much more clear-cut medical problems in situations at the very heart of scientific medicine. Garro's study (1994) of people with pain in the temporo-mandibular joint demonstrated how the experience of pain also involved culturally shared understandings of how the joint worked and their ideas and expectations about medicine. In particular, she notes the difficulty subjects had in managing the gap between their dominant cultural expectation that medicine should make one better and their continued pain, which made the pain harder to endure. Garro notes one respondent's question and response to the limitations of medical skill: ' "How long does it take to fix it?" Well, we may never fix it. That did it . . . The whole world changed. I just felt like I didn't belong here any more, I wasn't normal any more' (p. 78).

For this person, being normal had to do with being the sort of person whose illnesses can be cured by doctors. Even where there are observable physical illnesses or diseases, the process of expressing illness experience is embedded within a set of metaphors that must be understood within their cultural context in order to make sense of the patient's story.

Having identified something as wrong, nurses and other health care professionals try to organize people's problems so that they can do something about them. Murdach (1995) looked at the *heuristics* of social workers, that is, the informal rules they used to be able to cope. Pressure of work necessitated shortcuts. As one respondent said, 'In this place, we just have to use common sense in deciding things. It's nothing fancy. As soon as I come in the door, I have to get to work. Something's always happening – the phone's ringing or somebody wants something. I don't have time to think – I just act' (p. 756). Quick decision-making strategies involved dividing up a client's problems into three types:

(1) Immediate ones – risk of harm to self or others, for example suicide or threatening behaviour;
(2) Significant problems – difficulties with the law, housing and finances;
(3) Long-range problems, involving, for example, relationships, difficulties with employment or psychological development.

As Murdach says, these strategies were in accordance with a time-honoured heuristic in social work practice – namely to *partialize* the problem. By so doing, clinicians could focus their efforts and keep from being overwhelmed by the sheer unmanageableness of a rapidly unfolding chaotic situation (p. 754).

Thus, despite the metaphorical nature of clients' descriptions of their troubles, and despite the way in which their troubles are related to the culture and setting in which they are told, there is a curiously automatic quality to the way in which they are interpreted by health professionals. From Ndetei and Muhangi's (1979) conviction that their Kenyan patients must be suffering from depression or anxiety, to Murdach's (1995) social workers using their common sense to manage their workload, these interpretations are often immediate and intuitive. They make it look as if the problem or illness is out there, in the patient; they do not acknowledge that the problems have been organized and authored within an interpretive community of sufferers and carers.

SOCIAL SPACES OF SICKNESS: WHERE WE TELL OUR TROUBLES

Turner (1992) comments that 'Becoming sick requires the patient to learn how to perform according to certain norms of appropriate behaviour. There are appropriate and inappropriate rules of conduct which are expected of a person who has been correctly identified as "sick" ' (p. 215). Parsons' (1951) classic formulation of the role of the sick person involves four components: firstly that sick individuals are exempted from their normal social responsibilities; secondly that others accept that they cannot help being ill; thirdly that they should want to get well; and fourthly that they should seek appropriate medical help to enable their recovery (pp. 436–37). Gerhardt (1989) commented that the sick role is a kind of 'niche in the social system where the incapacitated may withdraw while attempting to mend their fences, with the help of the medical profession' (p. 15; see also Busfield, 1996). Being a good patient may even be about putting on a token show of healthiness – bearing up well, or being brave, for example.

More recently, researchers whose interest is in language have turned their attention to the accounts people give of their health. The categories of health and illness are not watertight: 'The healthy have much to say about their illness experience, while the sick are often at pains to show their "normality" ' (Radley and Billig, 1996, pp. 224–5). Telling stories about one's health, moreover, can be part of a complex conversational dance involving efforts at claiming that certain actions are sensible or permissible under the circumstances. This can be seen in an interview with a woman with rheumatoid arthritis reported by Williams (1993): ' "I'm not posh . . . but I'm comfortable. If anyone comes along and they don't like it . . . what can I do about it? I'm fortunate to keep it as straight as it is. If somebody's coming they take me as I am because doing too much I could cause myself a flare up. Why should I do it to cover something up? They must come in and find me as I am day today, which is right" ' (p. 99).

As Radley and Billig identify, this account contains elements of defensiveness and assertiveness, and has to be seen in the context of the difficulty the woman is having in caring for herself, her embarrassment at asking physiotherapists for help and not feeling able to appeal to her sons: 'The speaker is justifying her situation, thereby expressing the implied appropriateness of making such justifications . . . in giving her account, she asks for allowances to be made by the younger, healthy middle class, at-work, professionally sympathetic listener' (Radley and Billig, p. 226).

In the example above, the sufferer tells about her situation with very little guidance from the researcher. Many health interviews are much more structured and so limit the nature of troubles talk that can be entered into. Fox (1993) looked at surgical ward rounds when surgeons and other members of the medical team visit patients in their beds after their operations. Fox describes this as enabling surgeons to sustain claims that the surgery has been successful – not an easy thing to do as, after surgery, patients might well be in considerably more pain than when they came into hospital. Fox notes that 'Surgeons organise the discourse of their interactions with patients around three themes: physiology, wound condition and recovery/discharge. These themes are surgeon-centred, and are organised to deny patients access to the agenda of these encounters' (p. 16). Patients who ask questions can be seen as difficult. In Fox's study, a Miss F. asked, 'Can I take this mask off?' whilst she was being interrogated by the surgeon. The surgeon commented in an aside to the researcher, 'I said she was going to be a difficult patient' (p. 24).

Hospitals have often been taken by social scientists (Becker, 1993; Fox, 1993) to be a space where patients are controlled by staff using a particular kind of language. In some areas, however, staff and patients have been observed collaborating to sustain a particular formulation of the patients' troubles. Weijts, Houtkoop and Mullen (1993) looked at talk about sex in medical settings and found that, in Europe at least, the telling of sexual troubles is often conducted through euphemisms and omissions rather than direct references. Dutch doctors and patients refer to 'it', and 'down there'; terms like 'the event itself' and 'afterwards' are used to describe sex, without the nature of the 'event' being specified very closely.

KEEPING THE RECORD STRAIGHT: STRATEGIES FOR TAKING AND MAKING SENSE OF PATIENTS' NOTES

The way that nurses record information about patients in their care is very important because entries may come under close scrutiny. Introductory textbooks for nursing students suggest that patient records can and must reflect a real person and real events. The diligent professional is described as searching after truth by collecting information about patients. The truth is presumed to be that a single set of events underlies the incomplete and sometimes conflicting accounts that confront nurses when they open filing cabinets in clinical settings. Here is how one introductory textbook deals with the problem of case histories:

Essential facts of the past history may be missing and the chronology of life events may be muddled; it is also sometimes extraordinarily difficult to elicit accurate information, for example on periods of unemployment or on the reasons for prescribing or changing the dosage of medication or the effects of such changes. It is also well known that obtaining information covering long periods of time from the person concerned or from other informants can be highly problematic, particularly in the 'softer' areas of personal relationships, which are often coloured by subjective opinion; moreover, different informants give conflicting accounts since behaviour fluctuates over time and varies in different situations.

(Ekdawi and Conning, 1994, p. 39)

Here, the work which has to be done to establish the medico-nursing version of the patient's story is particularly visible. To make the records useful, nurses have to be active in filling in the gaps in the written account of the patient's story, joining the dots as it were. The goal of obtaining accurate information, the authors surmise, is hampered by subjective opinions, the individuality and unreliability of patients and the way in which details may be omitted from the records.

As long ago as 1967, Garfinkel and Bittner expressed their frustration that patients' records were often so incomplete as to be useless for research purposes (Garfinkel and Bittner, 1967). More recently Allen (1994) has commented, 'What seemed so clear at the time it was written may be barely legible, unbelievably incomplete and perhaps legally indefensible later' (p. 172).

Despite their incompleteness, records in clinical settings are often treated as if what they say is incontrovertible or beyond doubt. Oakley (1979) documented how a doctor was unwilling to admit a mother's ability to recall the size of her family when her answer contradicted his records. As with many bureaucratic procedures, record keeping in health care is about applying standard categories and routines to novel phenomena; it is about 'people processing' (Prottas, 1979). Clients may be typified as good or bad clients in the records (Kelly and May, 1982). Bowler (1995) describes how midwives writing in the medical records of women of South Asian descent living in southern England stereotyped them: 'Some midwives described the Asian women as not motherly, unmaternal. Conflict between Western and Asian ideologies of postnatal care . . . can be seen here . . . The women's behaviour was seen as abnormal as it did not conform to the prevailing (socially constructed, Western) model of motherhood' (Bowler, 1995, p. 40). Because there were a number of difficulties for the midwives in completing the records, not least because the women came from cultures where it was not customary to remember one's date of birth, the midwives typified the women as uncooperative or simple minded.

Making records and interpreting them involves considerably more than dealing with essential facts. Accounts of patients in their records incorporate judgements and values too. Unfortunately, although there is a large literature on doctor–patient interaction (e.g. Ong *et al.*, 1995), there is much less on nurse-patient interaction, and little is known about how these latter interactions are reformulated into health care records. However, the process of record keeping has been written about extensively in introductory textbooks and in the technical and professional literature in terms such as these: 'Pertinent, timely and accurate nursing documentation promotes consistency in client care and effective communication between nurses and other health team members' (Bernick and Richards, 1994, p. 203). The British house magazine of the nursing profession, the *Nursing Times*, counsels gravely, 'Accurate and comprehensive recording of information concerning patient care is an integral part of nursing' (Murdock, 1995, p. 22). Weiler (1994) insists that nursing records should be 'FACT': 'Factual, accurate, complete, and timely' (p. 31). The assumptions about the nursing process and language which are embedded in these quotes are that language can reflect reality comprehensively and accurately and that it is unproblematic to produce a factual account of nursing interactions with clients. In fact, there is a great deal more to documentation than this, and at best the language nurses use can convey only an incomplete and partial picture of what happens between professionals and patients.

The fundamental difficulty that nurses confront in documenting the patient encounter is to ensure that what the patient has to say is packaged in such a way as to be amenable to nursing documentation. Such documentation is, of course, proliferating and taking on new forms as links between medico-nursing records, health management systems, the supervision of care delivery, legal systems and legislation grow ever closer. Hence there is a drive towards scaling, rating and quantifying matters of concern. The use of sedation is a case in point; recording the patient's response to sedation on a scale is advocated by Clarke (1994) in relation to gastric investigations. This is not because the experience of sedation is inherently numerical, but because the logic that documentation of patients' responses to treatment is an important aspect of nursing care is universally applied. Within this framework, standardization is vital. With a problem such as appendicitis, it is reasonable to agree that the patient's condition should be monitored in a particular way and records made of when various treatments were given. However, such is the drive for standardization that some authors wrestle with the problem of standardizing much more complex areas of care such as those found in psychiatric nursing. Menneberg (1995) discusses attempts to standardize the process of psychiatric admission and care planning. Recording the softer aspects of care is also an important part of nursing documentation: 'Reassuring patients and their families when they're anxious, calming them when they're angry, helping them make choices and solve problems' (Jost, 1995, p. 46). If such interventions are not recorded, then, as Menneberg insists, 'You may not be getting the credit you deserve' (1995).

Here we see another factor in the proliferation of documentation – ensuring that the work of nurses is seen to count and thereby protecting jobs. It is in this context that Clark and Lang (1992) advocate the development of an international classification of nursing practice so as to 'Advance the knowledge necessary for cost effective delivery of quality nursing care' (p. 109). We are highly sceptical about the benefits of using standardized classifications of what nurses do. This is something we will discuss more fully towards the end of our book. Broadly, we consider such an approach to be totalitarian, controlling and ultimately impracticable. Most importantly, standardization limits what is at the heart of nursing – its diverse responses to the health needs of others, which themselves are constantly changing. Such excessive response to the need for greater clarity in nurse documentation is found elsewhere. Casey (1995) advocates that nurses themselves should be subject to regulation and supervision to encourage them to document patients' condition and to care more effectively. On the understanding that it is the job of nurses to provide information and education to the patient, Casey advocates formalizing what it is that nurses are supposed to teach and patients to learn on forms and flowsheets. This view suggests that nurses cannot be expected to become skilful, versatile and self-reflexive communicators. It is a view that we find deeply limited. In a similar guise we find Herbst (1992) insisting 'if you didn't write it down, it wasn't done'. This implies that a highly documented nursing system is one which makes it easier to secure compliance and ensure supervision and control.

A world of compliant patients and diligent note-taking nurses has always been the dream of managers. In what ways is the dream a nightmare? Ever since the early years of the twentieth century, social scientists (e.g. Weber, 1978) and managers have been interested in the ways in which the commitment of individuals to the organization's creeds might be increased. Record keeping helps secure the 'normative commitments' of subordinates to their superior's power (Witten, 1993) and enables organisations to 'dramatize their warrants to legitimacy' (Witten, 1993, p. 102). Looked at in this way, record keeping as a means of regulation and control takes on a rather sinister appearance, as it is about controlling the behaviour of nurses themselves as much as 'improving' their communication.

Foucault's classic study *Discipline and Punish* (1977) examines the role of regulation and supervision and finds that the more opportunity superiors have to observe the work of subordinates, the more subordinates will adhere to the procedures, policies and guidelines laid down. In the same way, records are a means of supervising patients, so it is not surprising that there is a link between more documentation and greater patient compliance. The power of written documentation is considerable and it is important to be aware of whether the compliance it secures from health care workers, such as nurses, and patients is working in the best interests of both.

THE DOMINANCE OF MEDICAL RECORDS OVER NURSING RECORDS

In many clinical settings, the records made by doctors are accorded a higher status than those made by nurses. The medical record is considered to define reality in a way that nursing records are not. Berg (1996) notes the powerful, central, constitutive and transformative role of medical records and shows how doctors include or exclude information that arises from the practitioner-patient relationship in a highly selective and elaborative way. Because the records exist as printed forms with predefined categories, they aid in the process of detailing the patients' problems in ways that are medically relevant. Summarizing reduces the unruly, unauthorized complexity of patients' talk of distress and imposes another, medically approved frame of reference. In settings where nurses have a more active authorial role, much of what Berg observes about the medical record's constitutive and organizational roles can be extended to the nursing record. Nursing keeps its own record which constitutes patient reality in its own terms and directs nursing action to deal with that reality.

Nurses, like doctors, may use reading the notes and writing in them to establish turn taking in the conversation of the therapeutic encounter. Looking at a client as he or she speaks and nodding can elicit more information than looking down and writing. In Berg's study, the manners of health care encounters seem to be that when the doctor looks at the patient expectantly it's their turn; when he looks down and writes, the patient's turn is over: 'His writing and reading as such are instrumental in the shaping of the way turns are distributed . . . Drawing a line beneath notes written down not only physically separates this entry from the rest: it is also a clear message that the consultation is over (especially when the physician also closes the patient's record)' (p. 508). The doctor reads and writes during the consultation; the patient does not. Thus the expert–client relationship is maintained. What emerges as a result of such reading and writing activity is patient compliance. In this view, language and authorship are vital for the business of doctoring or nursing. In order to be a patient, you first need to be defined as someone who has a problem the hospital can deal with, and then to be identified as someone sufficiently compliant that you can be treated.

One way of gaining insight into how records mediate the relationship between health professionals and patients is to imagine what would happen if all the records in all hospitals and health centres were to vanish overnight. Berg demonstrates that the record is not just an auxiliary feature of clinical life but that it is 'a material form of semi-public memory: relieving medical personnel's burden of organising and keeping track of the work to be done and its outcomes. The medical record is a structured distributing and collecting device, where all tasks concerning a patient's trajectory must begin and end. The simple ticking of a box, or the jotting down of some words set organisational routines in motion' (p. 510). What is striking about this description is the record's ability to 'set' hospital activity in motion. The medical record reinforces supervision: 'The availability of such an overviewable, durable and moveable set of inscriptions allows physicians the opportunity to extend their gaze across time and space. In other words, the record enables past and distant work – and spaces and time scales otherwise unimaginable – to be brought into the present' (p. 511). The records enable staff to make sense of their patients. Berg insists that 'The reality of a patient's body is assessed and transformed through layers of paperwork . . . The practices of reading and writing the record, then, are practices of reading and writing the patient's body; the practices of representation are indistinguishable from the activities they supposedly represent' (p. 511). Berg also sees the medical record as excluding nurses:

> The only information that the nurses enter into the medical record is what needs to be logged on the temperature chart. This form prestructures what data need to be collected, how, and how often. Blood pressure needs to be entered daily, while the temperature and pulse graph divides the 'day' into four eight-hour periods. Similarly the tabular format requires a highly standardised mode of entry: the effect of 'oversight in a quick glance' which this format affords is only achieved if nurses stick to reporting the fluid losses in millilitres and the drug dosages in a standard 'frequency times dosage' format. (p. 512)

The nursing text only enters the medical record here in a highly neutered, disempowered way. In contrast, 'The unstructured format of the case history forms creates responsibilities for physicians and affirms their position as the "central actor" in the structuring of the patient's trajectory' (p. 512). Berg's work suggests to nurses that they have to work hard to get their voices heard.

Berg effectively highlights the paper life of health care. The paper lives of doctors and nurses differ. Brevity is valued above discursiveness, but creates its own set of problems:

> The brevity and conciseness required for the record to work at the same time necessitates continuous 'repair work' . . . More generally, there is a continuous toing-and-froing between nurses, registrars and senior physicians about the very same records . . . What is true for the entries is also true for the structure of the form: the sections do not spell out how they are to be used. Their relevance often needs to be (re)assessed for the situation at hand: the organisational rules inscribed in the forms are constantly reinterpreted or overridden. (p. 514)

The records – medical or nursing – are public documents or repositories in which are stored the actions of professionals for inspection or auditing. Berg's critical scrutiny of medical records does not mean that he sees them as entirely false. Rather, he argues that they give an 'adequate rendering' (p. 519) that does the job of facilitating the clinic's business. He considers selectivity as vital for preservation of the record as organizational memory, a memory base which may be improved by computer technology (Dick and Steen, 1991). However, Berg believes that 'It makes sense to investigate just what type of memory a record embodies, what (links between) data are deemed more relevant than others, and what type of action or intervention it affords and what not' (p. 520).

Attempts to make sense of authorship in nursing include the work of Pridham and Schutz (1985), who state, 'If nursing is to make clear its contribution to health care, a language that is equal to the task is a necessity' (p. 122). They argue that nursing language should apply to all nursing disciplines, describe or characterize the nursing contribution, restrict itself to nursing issues, and accommodate the various nursing definitions of health and conceptual models of care. Finally, it should be 'Formulated in terms that are meaningful to and stated from the perspective of the individuals who present health-related problems to nurses' (p. 122).

This dream of a universal, user-friendly nursing language which can compete in the marketplace of health care has not yet been realized. Whether it can be or not, work such as Berg's highlights the struggle nurses have in many health care settings to gain some control over what is authored, or, indeed, what is deemed worthy of being read.

NEW TIMES, NEW RECORDS, NEW AUTHORSHIP

The circumstances under which records are made, the technology available to do it, and the purposes for which it is done are all subject to change and affect the authorship of the records themselves. Pressing keys to highlight boxes on a computer screen is very different from writing record entries in longhand. The opportunity to continue on a separate sheet or make notes on the back of a form is missing if the computer will accept only certain precoded answers.

Managers and service planners have attempted to increase the productivity of record takers by introducing computer-aided documentation systems (Olson, 1994). Despite some favourable reports that recording information in this way is faster and more comprehensive, the introduction of computers into care situations has not always been a success. Marr *et al.* (1993) studied nursing documentation following heavy investment in information technology at New York University Medical Center. Computer terminals placed next to patients' beds were scarcely used. However, some terminals that were located in rooms away from the patients were regularly used to make records. It could be speculated that this pattern of use might reflect the way that nurses tried to attend to patients in the nursing encounter rather than sit at the terminals and that filling in the records is something staff did in private so as to have a few moments' respite from the otherwise relentless interpersonal contact of hospital nursing.

There is now an assumption in the literature on nursing that the more documentation the better. The legal status of records has become prominent recently with nurses being urged to be aware that legal challenges to treatment and decision making may be mounted by patients and relatives (Weiler, 1994). In the USA, defensive documentation is advocated with a view to possible liability cases (Cummings, 1993). The relationship between documentation and care is made explicit by Christie (1993) in a study of new documentation in accident and emergency nursing: 'Overall, the documentation showed significant improvement. Therefore, it could be assumed that there had been an improvement in the quality of care' (p. 1758). Christie's argument that the more documentation there is, the more care there is, is naïve to say the least!

The drive towards documentation may leave many nurses lagging behind. Howse and Bailey (1992) highlight nurses' lack of confidence in their writing skills and their difficulty in articulating what exactly is done in nursing practice. Comprehensive, accurate recording of what is 'out there' in the patient is not likely to be achieved in nursing contexts, just as contemporary philosophers refute the notion that scientists can report an objective reality (Popper, 1959; Kuhn, 1962; Feyerabend, 1975). Indeed, studies of scientific reasoning (Gilbert and Mulkay, 1984), telling the truth (Nash, 1985) and telling factual accounts (Potter, 1996) suggest that there are a great many social rituals and linguistic devices involved in these apparently straightforward practices. Adding more detail suggests that the writer or speaker is trying to be convincing. It does not necessarily correspond to what you would have seen if you had been there in the first place. Therefore the drive towards accuracy and completeness can take us only so far. It is important to be aware of these limitations. Nurses who believe that documentation does not quite reflect what they do are in some ways philosophically sophisticated.

CONCLUSIONS

One response to the search for accuracy in records is to regard them as discursive – that is, constituted in and through language. Sacks (1972) counselled 'Be interested in what you've got' and what we have is language. As Harper (1996) argues, 'Mental health is an arena of discursive encounters, as indeed is physical health (Stainton-Rogers, 1991). Thinking about one's emotional state, discussing it with others, talking with one's general practitioner or other health professional are all textually constituted' (pp. 438–9). This applies to all disciplines of nursing.

Authoring in medical contexts is not just a matter of telling the story or writing the report. This chapter has shown how the language used is bound up with the conventions and genres of health care speech and writing and how cultural frames of reference give resources of meaning. Nursing works within a textually mediated reality such that the process of reading and writing is a key feature of medical and nursing encounters, and often the structure of the encounter between patient and professional is dictated by the filling in of records and making notes. Authoring is a dynamic part of the healing encounter.

In conclusion let us consider more fully what implications the issues here have for nursing. We hope to have generated some awareness of how complex and all-pervasive these issues are for speakers, writers, hearers and readers in health care settings. Most of us leave school knowing how to read and write but few of us are fully aware of the implications of these apparently simple activities. Nurses are involved in a complex linguistic dance and have been active in putting together the collage of ideas and images that make up health care. It is important to develop a systematic awareness of where these ideas and images come from and our own role in reconstructing them every time we speak or write.

Striving to have complete, accurate or even fully computerized records will bog the nursing profession down in a process which ultimately leaves it subordinate to doctors. Rather than simply failing at the hopeless task of making the records complete and accurate, nurses are in a unique position to shift the focus of language in such a way as to empower their own profession and their patients. Recognizing the generative or constructive work involved in authorship is one way of stepping into a new way of thinking about nursing and gives nurses a new measure of creative control over their contribution to the complex storytelling which goes on in health care settings. Through a greater awareness of the power of language to construct reality, nurses may choose to take a more critical look at the language they and other health professionals use. Indeed, they may become aware that delivering language is intimately bound up with delivering care. If nursing is going to have some say in its own future it must critically reflect upon its language and the language of other professionals and fight for the validity of nursing talk and writing. Most importantly, it will need to resist or become heretical about moves to standardize that language for them. Nurses must not assume that other nurses working to standardize what they communicate are on their side. They are not – they are fitting in all too snugly with wider political and economic fashions.

SUMMARY

Let us end this chapter by recapping some of the ground that we have covered. Authoring in medical contexts is not just a matter of telling the story or writing the report. We have shown how the language used is bound up with the conventions and genres of health care speech and writing, how there are cultural frames of reference at work which give us resources of meaning and ways of speaking so we can understand what is meant by, say, 'nerves' or, in the case of medical students at Kansas University, what a 'crock' is. Throughout this chapter we have emphasized how nursing works with a textually mediated reality. However, the way we speak about distress, from trying to make it look like we're bearing up well despite the pain, to cleaning up our act in front of people who might complain, is much more than the inert bundle of language that the term 'text' implies. We have tried to emphasize how important the stories of sickness are and the work that sufferers and staff in health care settings do to make sure that they are told these stories in the right way – that is, to ensure that they're told so as to facilitate the business of doctoring and nursing.

The process of authoring gets even more complex when we consider what happens when the records are written, reports made, referral letters composed and assessments completed. All this writing, judging by the complaints over the last 30 years, is often full of mistakes, omissions and inconsistencies. Many traditionally orientated authors have to work quite hard to keep a grip on the idea that there's a real patient there at all behind the confusion in many records. At the same time there is a growing concern that if the documentation is incomplete, then we won't get paid for the work we do.

As we have also argued, the process of reading and writing is a key feature of medical and nursing encounters and often the structure of the encounter between patient and professional is organized around filling in the records and making notes. Authoring, then, is a dynamic part of the healing encounter and something that nurses would be wise to spend some time reflecting upon.

REFERENCES

Allen, A. (1994) Does your documentation defend or discredit? *Journal of Post Anaesthesia Nursing*, 9(3), 172–3.

Allen, D.G. (1995) Hermeneutics: philosophical traditions and nursing practice research. *Nursing Science Quarterly*, 8(4), 174–82.

American Psychiatric Association (1994) *Diagnostic and Statistical Manual of Mental Disorders*, 4th edn (DSM-IV), American Psychiatric Association, Washington.

Barker, P.J. (1996) Chaos and the way of Zen: psychiatric nursing and the uncertainty principle. *Journal of Psychiatric and Mental Health Nursing*, 3, 235–43.

Becker, H.S. (1993) How I learned what a crock was. *Journal of Contemporary Ethnography*, 22(1), 28–35.

Becker, H.S. Geer, B. Hughes, E. and Strauss, A. (1961) *Boys in White*, University of Chicago Press, Chicago.

Bennett, N.A. Spoth, R.L. and Borgen, F.H. (1991) Bulimic symptoms in high school females: prevalence and relationship with multiple measures of psychological health. *Journal of Community Psychology*, 19(1), 13–28.

Bernick, L. and Richards, P. (1994) Nursing documentation: a program to promote and sustain development, *Journal of Continuing Education in Nursing*, 25(5), 203–8.

Bhatia, V.K. (1993) *Analysing Genre: Language Use in Professional Settings*, Longman, London.

Billig, M. (1989a) The argumentative nature of holding strong views: a case study. *European Journal of Social Psychology*, 19, 203–23.

Billig, M. (1989b) Psychology, rhetoric and cognition. *History of the Human Sciences*, 2, 289–307.

Bowler, I. (1995) Further notes on record taking and making in maternity care: the case of South Asian descent women. *Sociological Review*, 43(1), 36–51.

Boyle, M. (1990) *Schizophrenia: a scientific delusion*, Routledge, London.

Boyle, M. (1992) Form and content, function and meaning in the analysis of schizophrenic behaviour. *Clinical Psychology Forum*, 47, 10–15.

Boyle, M. (1994) Schizophrenia and the art of the soluble. *The Psychologist: Bulletin of the British Psychological Society*, 17, 399–404.

Bracken, P.J. (1993) Post empiricism and psychiatry: meaning and methodology in cross cultural research. *Social Science and Medicine*, 36(3), 265–72.

Burstow, B. (1992) *Radical Feminist Therapy: Working in the Context of Violence*, Sage, London.

Busfield, J. (1996) *Men, Women and Madness: Understanding Gender and Mental Disorder*, Macmillan, London.

Carr, J.E. and Vitaliano, P.P. (1985) The theoretical implications of converging research on depression and the culture bound syndromes, in *Culture and Depression* (eds A. Kleinman and B. Good), University of California Press, Los Angeles.

Casey, F.S. (1995) Documenting patient education: a literature review. *Journal of Continuing Education in Nursing*, 26(6), 257–60.

Castro, R. (1995) The subjective experience of health and illness in Ocuituco: a case study. *Social Science and Medicine*, 41(7), 1005–21.

Chesters, L. (1994) Women's talk: food, weight and body image. *Feminism and Psychology*, 4(3), 449–57.

Christie, J. (1993) Does the use of an assessment tool in the accident and emergency department improve the quality of care? *Journal of Advanced Nursing*, 18(11), 1758–71.

Clark, J. and Lang, N. (1992) Nursing's next advance: an internal. *International Nursing Review*, 39(4), 109–12.

Clarke, B.A. (1994) A new approach to assessment and documentation of conscious sedation during endoscopic examination. *Gastroenterology Nursing*, 16(5), 199–203.

Clarke, L. (1996) The last post? Defending nursing against the postmodernist maze. *Journal of Psychiatric and Mental Health Nursing*, 3, 257–65.

Crisp, A.H. (1980) *Anorexia Nervosa: Let Me Be*, Grune and Stratton, New York.

Cummings, C.M. (1993) *Defensive Documentation: A Line of Defense*. Video distributed by American Journal of Nursing Company, New York.

Curt, B. (1994) *Textuality and Tectonics*, Open University Press, Buckingham.

Dally, P., Gomez, J. and Isaacs, A.J. (1979) *Anorexia Nervosa*, Heinemann, London.

Darbyshire, P. (1994) Reality bites: the theory and practice of nursing narratives. *Nursing Times*, 90(40), 31–3.

Dick, R.S. and Steen, E.B. (1991) *The Computer Based Patient Record: An Essential Technology for Health Care*, National Academy Press, Washington DC.

Edwards, D. and Potter, J. (1992) *Discursive Psychology*, Sage, London.

Ekdawi, M. Y. and Conning, A.M. (1994) *Psychiatric Rehabilitation: A Practical Guide*, Chapman & Hall, London.

Fairclough, N. (1989) *Language and Power*, Longman, London.

Fenton, S. and Sadiq-Sangster, A. (1996) Culture, relativism, and the expression of mental distress: South Asian women in Britain. *Sociology of Health and Illness*, 18(1), 66–85.

Feyerabend, P. (1975) *Against Method*, New Left Books, London.

Fish, S. (1980) *Is There a Text in This Class? The Authority of Interpretive Communities*, Harvard University Press, Cambridge, MA.

Foucault, M. (1965) *Madness and Civilisation*, Random House, New York.

Foucault, M. (1975) *The Birth of the Clinic: An Archaeology of Medical Perception*, Vintage, New York.

Foucault, M. (1977) *Discipline and Punish: The Birth of the Prison* (trans. A. Sheridan), Penguin, Harmondsworth.

Fox, N.J. (1993) Discourse, organisation and the surgical ward round. *Sociology of Health and Illness*, 15(1), 16–42.

Garfinkel, H. and Bittner, E. (1967) Good organizational reasons for bad clinic records, in *Studies in Ethnomethodology* (ed. H. Garfinkel), Prentice Hall, New York.

Geertz, C. (1983) *Local Knowledge: Further Essays in the Interpretation of Culture*, Basic Books, New York.

Gelder, M., Gath, D. and Mayou, R. (1994) *Concise Oxford Textbook of Psychiatry*, Oxford University Press, Oxford.

Gerhardt, U. (1989) *Ideas about Illness: An Intellectual and Political History of Medical Sociology*, Macmillan, London.

Gilbert, G.N. and Mulkay, M. (1984) *Opening Pandora's Box: A Sociological Analysis of Scientists' Discourse*, Cambridge University Press, Cambridge.

Goffman, E. (1981) *Forms of Talk*, Blackwell, Oxford.

Gorna, R. (1996) *Vamps, Virgins and Victims: How Can Women Fight AIDS?* Cassell, London.

Gottleib, M.S. (1981) Pneumocystis carnii pneumonia and mucosal candidiasis in previously healthy homosexual men. Evidence of a new acquired cellular immunodeficiency. *New England Journal of Medicine*, 305(24), 1425–31.

Gramsci, A. (1971) *Prison Notebooks* (trans. Q. Hoare and G. Nowell-Smith), Lawrence & Wishart, London.

Griffith, H.M. and Robinson, K.R. (1993) Current procedural terminology (CPT) code services provided by nurse specialists. *Image: Journal of Nursing Scholarship*, 25(3), 178–86.

Gull, W.W. (1874) Anorexia nervosa. *Transactions of the Clinical Society of London*, 7.

Hall, S., Critcher, C., Jefferson, T. *et al.* (1978) *Policing the Crisis: Mugging, the State and Law and Order*, Macmillan, London.

Harper, D.J. (1992) Defining delusion and the serving of professional interests, *British Journal of Medical Psychology*, 65, 357–69.

Harper, D.J. (1994) Histories of suspicion in a time of conspiracy. *History of the Human Sciences*, 7, 89–109.

Harper, D.J. (1996) Deconstructing 'paranoia': Towards a discursive understanding of apparently unwarranted suspicion. *Theory and Psychology*, 6(3), 423–48.

Hawes, L. (1977) Towards a hermeneutic phenomenology of communication. *Communication Quarterly*, 25, 30–41.

Herbst, L. (1992) *If You Didn't Write It Down It Wasn't Done: Documentation in Home Health Nursing*. Video distributed by American Journal of Nursing Company, New York.

Hollinger, R. (1994) *Postmodernism and the Social Sciences*, Sage, London.

Howse, E. and Bailey, J. (1992) Resistance to documentation: a nursing research issue. *International Journal of Nursing Studies*, 29(4), 371–81.

Hulme, P. (1996) Everybody means something: collaborative conversation explored. *Changes*, 14, 67–72.

Jost, K.E. (1995) Psychosocial care: document it. *American Journal of Nursing*, 95(7), 46–9.

Kelly, M.P. and May, D. (1982) Good and bad patients: a review of the literature and theoretical critique. *Journal of Advanced Nursing*, 7, 147–56.

Kitzinger, C. (1986) Introducing and developing Q as a feminist methodology: a study of accounts of lesbianism, in *Feminist Social Psychology* (ed. S. Wilkinson), Open University Press, Milton Keynes.

Kitzinger, C. and Perkins, R. (1993) *Changing Our Minds*, Onlywomen Press, London.

Kitzinger, J. (1993) Sexual violence and compulsory heterosexuality, in *Heterosexuality: A Feminism and Psychology Reader* (eds S. Wilkinson and C. Kitzinger), Sage, London.

Kiviniemi, K. (1994) Conscious awareness and memory during general anaesthesia. *AANA Journal*, 62(5), 441–9.

Kleinman, A. (1987) Anthropology and psychiatry: the role of culture in cross cultural research on illness. *British Journal of Psychiatry*, 151, 447–54.

Kronemeyer, R. (1980) *Overcoming Homosexuality*, Macmillan, New York.

Kuhn, T.S. (1962) *The Structure of Scientific Revolutions*, University of Chicago Press, Chicago.

Lacan, J. (1977) *The Four Fundamental Concepts of Psychoanalysis*, Hogarth, London.

Authorship

Lakoff, G. (1987) *Women, Fire and Dangerous Things: What Categories Reveal about the Mind*, University of Chicago Press, Chicago.

Lemert, C. (1990) The uses of French structuralisms in sociology, in *Frontiers of Social Theory: The New Syntheses* (ed. G. Ritzer), Columbia University Press, New York.

Lindlof, T. (1988) Media audiences as interpretive communities. *Communication Yearbook*, 11, 81–107

Lyotard, J.-F. (1984) *The Postmodern Condition*, University of Minnesota Press, Minneapolis.

Marr, P.B., Duthie, E., Glassman, K.S. *et al.* (1993) Bedside terminals and quality of nursing documentation. *Computers in Nursing*, 11(4), 176–82.

Martin, J.R. (1984) Language, register and genre, in *Children Writing: A Reader* (ed. J.R. Martin), Deakin University Press, Geelong, Victoria.

Menneberg, S.R. (1995) Standards of care in documentation of psychiatric care. *Clinical Nurse Specialist*, 9(3), 142–8.

Moscovici, S. (1984) The phenomenon of social representations, in *Social Representations* (eds R.M. Farr and S. Moscovici), Cambridge University Press, Cambridge.

Mulkay, M. and Gilbert, G.N. (1985) Opening Pandora's box: a new approach to the sociological analysis of theory choice. *Knowledge and Society*, 5, 113–39.

Murdach, A.D. (1995) Clinical practice and heuristic reasoning. *Social Work*, 40(6), 752–8.

Murdock, D. (1995) Careful recording. *Nursing Times*, 91(47), 44–5.

Nash, J. (1985) *Social Psychology: Society and Self*, West Publishing Co., St Paul, MN.

Ndetei, D.M. and Muhangi, J. (1979) The prevalence and clinical presentation of psychiatric illness in a rural setting in Kenya. *British Journal of Psychiatry*, 135, 269–72.

Oakley, A. (1979) *Becoming a Mother*, Martin Robertson, London.

Olson, L.L. (1994) Commentary on voice activated nursing documentation: on the cutting edge. *Aone's Leadership Perspectives*, 2(1), 14.

Ong, L.M.L., de Haes, J.C.J., Hoos, A.M. and Lammes, F.B. (1995) Doctor–patient communication: a review of the literature. *Social Science and Medicine*, 40(7), 903–18.

Parsons, T. (1951) *The Social System*, Routledge & Kegan Paul, London.

Patel, V. and Winston, M. (1994) 'Universality of mental illness' revisited: assumptions, artefacts and new directions. *British Journal of Psychiatry*, 165, 437–40.

Perkins, R. (1996) Combating anti-lesbianism in mental health. *Women and Mental Health Forum*, 1, 16–21.

Polivy, J. and Herman, P. (1987) The diagnosis and treatment of normal eating. *Journal of Consulting and Clinical Psychology*, 55, 635–44.

Popper, K. (1959) *The Logic of Scientific Discovery*, Hutchinson, London.

Potter, J. (1996) *Representing Reality: Discourse, Rhetoric and Social Construction*, Sage, London.

Pridham, K.F. and Schutz, M.E. (1985) Rationale for a language for naming problems from a nursing perspective. *Image: The Journal of Nursing Scholarship*, 17(4), 122–7.

Prottas, J.M. (1979) *People-processing*, Lexington Books, Lexington, MA.

Psathas, G. (1995) *Conversation Analysis*, Sage, Thousand Oaks, CA.

Radley, A. and Billig, M. (1996) Accounts of health and illness: dilemmas and representations. *Sociology of Health and Illness*, 18(2), 230–40.

Radway, J. (1984) *Reading the romance*, University of North Carolina Press, Chapel Hill.

Rand, C.S. and Kuldau, J.M. (1992) Epidemiology of bulimia nervosa in a general population: Sex, age, race and socioeconomic status. *International Journal of Eating Disorders*, 11(1), 37–44.

Ricouer, P. (1977) *The Rule of Metaphor: Multi-disciplinary Studies of the Creation of Meaning in Language* (trans. R. Czerny, K. McLaughlin and J. Costello), University of Toronto Press, Toronto.

Ritzer, G. (1992) *Sociological Theory*, McGraw Hill, New York.

Russell, G. (1979) Bulimia nervosa: an ominous variant of anorexia nervosa. *Psychological Medicine*, 9(3), 429–48.

Sachs, L. (1983) *Evil Eye or Bacteria: Turkish Migrant Women and Swedish Health Care, Stockholm Studies in Social Anthropology*, University of Stockholm, Stockholm.

Sacks, H. (1972) An initial investigation into the usability of conversational data for doing sociology, in *Studies in Social Interaction* (ed. D. Sudnow), Free Press, New York.

Sartorius, N., Shapiro, R. and Jablonsky, A. (1974) The International Pilot Study of Schizophrenia. *Schizophrenia Bulletin*, 2, 21–35.

Shotter, J. (1993) *The Cultural Politics of Everyday Life*, Open University Press, Buckingham.

Sontag, S. (1979) *Illness as Metaphor*, Allen Lane, London.

Stainton-Rogers, W. (1991) *Explaining Health and Illness: An Exploration of Diversity*, Harvester Wheatsheaf, Hemel Hempstead.

Stevenson, C. (1996) The Tao, social constructivism and psychiatric nursing practice and research. *Journal of Psychiatric and Mental Health Nursing*, 3, 217–24.

Swales, J.M. (1990) *Genre Analysis*, Cambridge University Press, Cambridge.

Taylor, I. and Robertson, A. (1994) A sensitive question. *Nursing Times*, 90, 51.

Turner, B.S. (1992) *Regulating Bodies: Essays in Medical Sociology*, Routledge, London.

Ventola, E. (1988) Text analysis in operation, in *New Developments in Systematic Linguistics*, vol. 2 (eds R.P. Fawcett and D. Young), Pinter Publications, London.

Weber, M. (1978) *Economy and Society* (trans. G. Roth and C. Wittich) University of California Press, Berkeley.

Weijts, W., Houtkoop, H. and Mullen, P. (1993) Talking delicacy: speaking about sexuality during gynaecological consultations. *Sociology of Health and Illness*, 15(3), 295–314.

Weiler, K. (1994) Legal aspects of nursing documentation for the Alzheimer's patient. *Journal of Gerontological Nursing*, 20(4), 31–40.

Williams, G.H. (1993) Chronic illness and the pursuit of virtue in everyday life, in Radley, A. (Ed.) *Worlds of Illness: Biographical and Cultural Perspectives in Health and Disease* (ed. A. Radley) Routledge, London.

Willis, P. (1980) Notes on method, in *Culture, Media, Language* (eds S. Hall, D. Hobson, C. Lowe and P. Willis) Hutchinson, London.

Witten, M. (1993) Narrative and the culture of obedience at the workplace, in *Narrative and Social Control: Critical Perspectives* (ed. D.K. Mumby), Sage, Thousand Oaks, CA.

Wooffitt, R. (1992) *Telling Tales of the Unexpected*, Harvester Wheatsheaf, Brighton.

World Health Organisation (1992) *The ICD-10 Classification of Mental and Behavioural Disorders: Cultural Descriptions and Diagnostic Guidelines*, World Health Organisation, Geneva.

KEY REFERENCES

Berg, M. (1996) Practices of reading and writing: the constitutive role of the patient record in medical work. *Sociology of Health and Illness*, 18(4), 499–524.

Cheek, J. and Rudge, T. (1994) Nursing as textually mediated reality. *Nursing Inquiry*, 1(1), 15–22.

Garro, L. (1994) Narrative representations of chronic illness experience: cultural models of illness, mind and body in stories concerning the temporo-mandibular joint (TMJ). *Social Science and Medicine*, 38(6), 775–88.

Migliore, S. (1993) 'Nerves': the role of metaphor in the cultural framing of experience. *Journal of Contemporary Ethnography*, 22(3), 331–60.

Proctor, A., Morse, J.M. and Khonsari, E.S. (1996) Sounds of comfort in the trauma center: how nurses talk to patients in pain. *Social Science and Medicine*, 42(12), 1669–80.

3 COMMUNICATION: HOW DO WE TELL?

AIMS

This chapter aims to raise awareness of how the form of communication can influence what is said or written in health care contexts. Specifically, it aims to encourage appreciation of how language in health care has a distinctive quality. We intend to show that the *form* of how stories are told about people's problems tends to gear the nurse and other health professionals to the solutions that are available in the health care system.

We demonstrate how writing about clients is shaped by proximal features, like the structure of the recording form, and distal features like sociocultural beliefs. We establish the complex formal nature of written communication and show how this contrasts with the interactive, informal nature of spoken communication.

Finally, we make a plea for nurses to reflect more on the nature of the language they and other health care professionals use and how incautious language may entrap the very people health workers are trying to help.

INTRODUCTION: GENRES, REGISTERS OR LANGUAGE STYLES, AND SPECIFIC PURPOSES

A great deal of the caring work of nursing is accomplished and mediated through spoken and written language or, as Cheek and Rudge (1994) put it, nursing is a 'textually mediated reality'. They argue that much of nursing theory and practice is determined by how it is written about and described in policy documents, research papers and professional articles. If we consider language as a powerful social practice (Fairclough, 1989), or indeed as a 'loaded weapon' (Bolinger, 1980), it is vital that more research is carried out on the speech and writing produced and used in nursing to uncover the way nursing language exerts power within the constraints of its own genre or style and within the broader set of power relations that exist between doctors, nurses and patients (Fisher, 1995; Shotter, 1997). To do this, firstly we are faced with the mammoth task of simply trying to describe what goes on in institutional and community settings. Yet in order to make sense of what goes on, description is necessary for us to interpret and explain language use (Fairclough, 1989, p. 109).

Let us for a moment consider what languages we might find in clinical settings in Europe and North America. Certainly, there is a great deal of overlap between language in hospital or community care and language in general. However, it is possible to argue that language in nursing forms a specific genre or style of speech and writing. It is an organized social practice that does far more than simply reflect real objects or phenomena. It constructs reality. The simplest example of this is the transformation effected by referring to people as 'patients'. The term 'patient' will change the way the people see themselves and others see them. In this sense, language can be seen as a construction yard (Potter, 1996). Or, to put this in a health care context, perhaps we could see professional language as something more like an operating theatre. Language is an important tool in constructing the 'textually mediated realities' within which professionals work. There are important features that distinguish the kinds of language used in different contexts.

Key reference

As discussed in chapters 1 and 2, literary scholars and film critics have long been concerned with the concept of 'genre'. A genre involves a set of conventions as to the goals, purposes and communicative style of any language event. Often the term is used when referring to various kinds of literature and films, for example, tragedy, comedy, western, detective, romance and so on. But more recent definitions stress how the term can be applied more widely. For example Martin (1984, p. 25) says that 'a genre is a staged, goal oriented purposeful activity in which speakers engage as members of our culture . . . Virtually everything we do involves you participating in one or other genre.' Other authors have begun to identify some of the distinctive features of language in health settings. For example, as we discussed earlier, Proctor *et al.* (1996) identify the 'comfort talk register' – a kind of talk used by nurses dealing with patients in a US 'trauma center' which seemed to be to encourage patients to hold on and endure the situation a little longer.

One interesting way in which the issue of language use in professional contexts has been thought of is in terms of 'language for specific purposes' (Gunnarson, Nordberg and Linell, 1997). Here, scholars look at what people are doing with the language – communicating about patients, providing care, or offering comfort as in the example of the trauma centre above. At the same time, professional genres, registers or styles of language may just as easily set up barriers to communication (Wodak, 1996). That is, they may reduce the communicative possibilities between clients and professionals. Moreover, despite their appearances of precision and technical mastery, professional languages do not necessarily mean that professionals understand each other or that they are communicating more precisely, as we shall argue later.

The genre of nursing is further complicated by the constraints operating upon it, from the fear of being sued later to the design of the forms on which patients' details are recorded. In this chapter we will explore in more detail how communication in nursing settings has a distinctive form. This will be done by looking at three main examples. The first is a study of our own which examined the kind of writing about patients which nursing students performed; the second is taken from nursing records about people suffering from anxiety; and the third explores differences between the written and oral communication employed by nurses in an attempt to reorganize the delivery of hospital care.

FACT CONSTRUCTION: NURSING LANGUAGE AS AN 'OPERATING THEATRE'

The business of professionals using language to construct realities is not unique to nursing. Every workplace has a construction yard where its language, with its definitions, typifications and versions of reality, is put together. Nursing, we suggested above, can be thought of as having an 'operating theatre' of language. Looking at the parallels between the operations nurses perform on language and the work other professions do can be instructive. Romero (1986, p. 72) notes how journalists freely construct reality by controlling and shaping 'soft and vague' words that make up the 'facts': 'From the exercise of this freedom, and from such influences on his decisions as habit, ideology, and his understanding of what readers want, come the facts that we conventionally accept as such in the press.'

Like journalism, nursing involves a range of processes whereby facts about patients are arranged for a particular readership according to particular conventions. The nurse observes the complexity of patients' pains, illnesses and distress and uses a variety of professional routines and tacit or unstated theories about what has happened and what matters to construct a textual account.

In this chapter we shall firstly attempt to detect some quantitative evidence that the language of mental health nursing is distinctive, and therefore consolidate our claim that the various nursing desciplines obey generic conventions. Before we do this, however, let us remind ourselves why this is an important issue for nurses generally.

It is important because we aim to 'help increase consciousness of how language contributes to the domination of some people by others, because consciousness is the first step towards emancipation' (Fairclough, 1989, p. 1). Nursing language has long been ignored as a site of the use and abuse of power. In examining this area we aim to continue a process that we have begun elsewhere (Crawford, Nolan and Brown, 1995) to discover aspects of nursing practice that are in need of reform. Medico- nursing accounts of individuals are rarely subjected to critical analysis. Instead, medico-nursing files act as 'corporate biographies' which last into the future, and may entrap or incarcerate the patient just as effectively as any legal, physical or pharmacological constraint. Whereas they are perceived by those who write and use them as authoritative, we have argued that all too often they fictionalize and ultimately 'linguistically incarcerate' individuals. In line with many other scholars of language in work settings (e.g. Encandela, 1991; Boden, 1994), we believe that the language of reports and records reflects broader social relations, structures of authority, and communities of sense making. It is vital that those structures with which information is communicated are scrutinized, especially since language use is fundamental to professional practices of classifying, labelling and

Example 1

resolving clients' health problems in terms of existing categories. We have coined the term 'firing paper bullets' for the problematic aspects of professional communication which may work against the patient. This is a term to which we shall return in the discussion that follows. Professionals, though attempting to base their work on science and ethical reasoning, all too frequently invest or influence decision making with many of their own values and preferences.

EXAMPLE 1: NURSING STUDENTS MAKING SENSE OF 'DEPRESSION'

Our first example concerns an investigation of nursing students describing a depressed person. This is an important area of enquiry because students, as part of their learning process and professional socialization, are trying on their new 'linguistic uniforms'. Thus, the practices they use to speak and write in the appropriate genre might be particularly visible. Making written reports about individuals with health problems, not least those of a mental health nature, is central to nursing practice. These reports become part of a biographical file of the individual client, communicating assessments, plans, interventions and evaluations across time and between a variety of agents or services in different locations. Yet such reports or texts have all too often been interpreted transparently as truth bearing. Increasingly, discourse analysts are turning their attention to how telling stories about reality involves an array of linguistic devices to make our accounts persuasive, believable and convincing (Potter, 1996; Wooffitt, 1992). Language that claims to tell us about reality is meticulously organized in terms of style and vocabulary. As Harvey Sacks would have it, there is 'order at all points' (as quoted in Psathas, 1995). It is therefore our intention to present some evidence about the representations of patients constructed by nursing students. The student nurses were instructed to make their reports about patients in a way that paralleled report writing in professional practice. We shall use this information from students as a way of structuring the first part of this chapter. This will highlight several things.

Firstly, it will give us some information about the way students write as they work their way into the genre of nursing language. Secondly, it will give some structure to the comments we shall make about the existing literature on the subject. The features of students' language which we isolate provide a framework into which a good deal of the other scholarship on the issue can be slotted. Finally, it will enable us to make some recommendations about how the practice of making mental health nursing reports may be changed for the better and alert other nursing disciplines to the need for greater understanding and vigilance about their own report practices. Admittedly, our first example cannot do justice here to the various kinds of nursing reports, such as those constructed by general nurses, midwives, health visitors, and so on, but it does get the ball rolling. The hope is that other studies will fill in the gaps that we leave.

The data provided by nursing students, then, are not intended to form an exhaustive account of their use of language, nor are we arguing that a single description of language is appropriate in all situations. However, we shall highlight some shared features across their texts; some differences between the language used in nursing compared to the English language in general; some differences between individual writers; and discrepancies between nursing students' accounts and those of their qualified counterparts.

To date the whole issue of how exactly nurses textualize their observations and judgements has largely remained submerged and unexplored. In performing this study we aimed to examine what it is exactly that a particular group of nursing students write. Perhaps in the future, with the development of nursing as a degree level subject and the growing interest of scholars including ourselves in this area, we might see more focus on language in nurse education and research. Perhaps we will even see the development of 'textual management' courses for all nursing disciplines.

The genre of nursing reports revealed through word frequencies

In our study 26 nursing students were asked to observe a ten-minute video in which a person (the 'subject') described the nature of his problems to a psychiatrist. This was followed by a written task where they were instructed to make a judgement as to whether they would recommend this patient for hospitalization and indicate their main observations and reasons for their decision.

The analysis of reports that students produced in response to this task firstly involved producing a quantitative account of the way students used words in writing about the subject and comparing this with existing databases of the English language which have been compiled. Secondly, an analysis of the semantic features of the language used in the reports was undertaken. This included an examination of modal or modifying terms; terms used for the client; semantic sets that the participants drew upon; binomial expressions; stylistic features such as lexical density and the use of reported speech; and comparisons between student and qualified participants. The purpose of this exercise was to elicit from the students the types of words they used to describe the patient's condition and the reasoning behind their decisions.

To deal with the first feature of the students' accounts – their use of words – our investigation began with an examination of vocabulary frequency. We also distinguished between lexical and grammatical items in the body of text or 'corpus' produced by the nurses. Lexical items are words that carry content in language and are represented by the word classes: noun, verb, adjective, adverb and pronoun. Grammatical items are words that cement terms together in language and are represented by the word classes: preposition, conjunction, auxiliary verb, article and negative. In the discussion that follows we will be concentrating especially on the lexical items.

Example 1

The words used by the nursing students immediately gave a flavour of their point of origin. Perhaps it comes as no great surprise that the most common term was *he*, referring to the person, with *him* and *himself* also appearing frequently. Rather more interesting was a clutch of terms that were used several times by most students which included *depressed* and *depression*, as well as the more colloquial or ordinary *down* and *low*. The consequences of this were reflected in the frequent appearance of terms like *suicide* and *harm*. There were also a number of well-used expressions relating to the processes that might be gone through, for example *hospitalization*, *therapy* and *counselling*.

This distribution of terms immediately suggests the content of the texts and locates them as mental health nursing reports. This fact alone is a significant example of the power of lexical analysis to convey information about the dominant stylistic or generic features of texts. The most frequent lexical items used by the students were nouns: *life*, *family*, *depression*, *hospital*, *patient*. Furthermore, the two most frequent adjectives being *depressed* and *trapped* along with the pronoun *he* enables us to tie down the content even more specifically. These clues help us to infer quite confidently that the collection of words originated from a mental health care context.

Thus, from the frequency of lexical items in the material we have some evidence for the distinctive nature of the genre, register or style that the students are participating in when making these reports. Even at an early stage in their training, the students are trying on the uniform of professional language. This is partly determined by the task and subject matter to hand, yet there is a more generally recognizable quality to their choice of vocabulary. Furthermore, there are implications for practice embedded in these findings. An examination of the most frequent items in our corpus (body of writings) indicates that a protocol for language use could be designed to guide future report-making practice, not just in mental health nursing but in other nursing disciplines as well. If nursing language obeys generic conventions it is important for nurse educators to be aware of these so curricula for students can be designed and developed in order to better protect clients' interests. Clearly, 'redesigning' language is a contentious issue, but a move towards minimizing inaccuracies, irrelevancies and negative, judgemental terms is vital. This is no mere academic exercise, because what is said and written about clients has far-reaching implications (Crawford, Nolan and Brown, 1995). Overdosing clients' records with judgemental terms may be just as toxic as overdosing them on medication. Moreover, the awareness gained from a thorough examination of language practice will yield more descriptive accuracy, and encourage nurses to reflect critically on their use of language. As we shall discuss later, this does not mean we are in favour of standardizing nursing language. We prefer to promote a focus on the reflective abilities of individual nurses to scrutinize, monitor and change their language for the better.

Secondly, a number of items that were heavily used by students were repeated in different forms. For example, if we look at a set of words with a similar theme or base, for example *feel/feels/feeling/felt* and the item *feelings*, the combined frequencies rise to a level that would put them in the top ten of the most frequently used words. This is intriguing because in the English language in general, grammatical items such as 'the', 'of' 'and' and 'to' are the most common. As such, the register-specific nature of the references to 'feeling' in terms of what the interviewer *feels* or thinks and the interviewee *feels* or experiences strongly suggests a humanistic and client-centred approach to mental health nursing. However, the wide use of 'feeling' words may also heavily and indeed powerfully limit the space into which clients' problems can unfold and be understood.

Fortunately, the frequency of words in the English language has been the subject of extensive previous research. To compare the word frequency in the texts produced by the nursing students more formally with English in general, we used two extensive databases: the COBUILD Corpus (CC) and the Bank of English (BoE). In both of these large databases the top 20 places are filled almost exclusively by grammatical items rather than lexical items, such as *the*, *of*, *to* and *and*.

If we now look further at the most frequent words used by the students and the most frequently used words in the sample of 120 million words of the CC and BoE, we can make some further observations. Importantly, a number of the words that were used heavily by the nursing students are by no means as frequent in English as a whole. These are: *his*, *this*, *not*, *him*, *has*, and *feel*. The terms thus highlight the way that language in this context is about someone else – the patient. Thus, we have some evidence for the 'out-thereness' that is constructed in factual language (Potter, 1996, p. 150) as authors develop persuasive accounts of nature in scientific or psychiatric discourse.

There are some additional quantitative features that can be understood as part of the genre, register and topic of the texts produced by student nurses. For example *needs* is the most prominent verb after *feel*. This item is at the core of the meaning and function of the nursing texts and infers a strong focus on assessment of the individual's requirements, for example, 'The patient needs hospitalisation', or on his state of mind: 'The needs of the patient are many.' Again, the properties on which the assessment is based are fundamentally constructed and inferred as being a property of the patient. Although the diagnoses arrived at borrow heavily from psychiatric terminology, the participants are also venturing 'under the skull' into vocabularies of intra-psychic constructs of motivation and emotion to explain the patient's behaviour (Garfinkel, 1967; Potter and Wetherell, 1987).

Built-in uncertainty: are students hedging their bets?

A further prominent feature of reports generated by students was how they seemed to be uncertain about what it was they were conveying. That is, there is a high frequency of modal terms: *may*, *would*, *could*, *can*, *can't*, *should*, *will*, *might*. There are also two prominent modal

Example 1

verbs: *appears*, *seems*. Modality is concerned with possibility, prob-
ability, likelihood or intention. Latour and Woolgar (1986) describe
what they call a 'hierarchy of modalization' where high-modality
factual statements contrast with low-modality uncertainty, guesses and
possibility. That is, a high-modality statement like 'He showed some
significant signs of depression' is altogether more definite than 'He
seemed to be showing feelings of despair'. Of the terms generated by
the students, *may*, *might*, *appears* and *seems* are more sceptical – or
of lower modality – than *would, could, can, can't, should* and *will*.
Significantly, *may* has the greatest frequency. There are two possible
inferences that can be made from these features. One suggestion is
that the student group is uncertain in its assessments and oscillates
between indecisive and decisive statements. A second inference is
based on the notion that these modal statements are a feature of
academic language and are adopted by the students as part of doing
a classroom exercise. In a sense, they are pushing their descriptions
down the 'hierarchy of modalization' (see also Potter, 1996). Whilst
showing they are aware of the qualities of the patient and the
hospitalization and treatment possibilities, they are also forestalling
potential conflicts with other possible interpretations on the part of
the researchers. For example, one student wrote, 'It is questionable
whether at the moment he is using his diagnosis as mentally ill as an
excuse to not cope, maybe because he's scared to put the effort into
coping again.' Here, the writer is showing that she is able to entertain
speculations about the client's state of mind and inner workings but
at the same time showing the reader that she is aware that they are
speculations.

This feature of modalization has somewhat controversially been
noted as a feature of the language of disempowered groups (e.g.
Lakoff, 1975), and fits in with the position of nurses in hospital
hierarchies (Boden, 1994; Fisher, 1995). The relatively high rate of
use of modalizing terms may also be thought of as a way that nurses
hedge their bets. As Hewitt and Stokes (1975, p. 3) note, this is part   **Key reference**
of a strategy to 'ward off and defeat in advance doubts and negative
typifications which might result from intended conduct'. In other
words, highly hedged language is rather sophisticated as it anticipates
a variety of possible consequences and does not prematurely commit
the writer to a course of action which might prove contentious later.
In this sense perhaps our participants are not so much firing paper
bullets as firing blanks – avoiding committing themselves to any
position or viewpoint. They use language which is so hedged as to
reduce its potential for enabling action. At the same time they are able
to express that they are sophisticated thinkers about the human
condition and can fill in what they see to be missing. For example,
one participant writes, 'I don't think he is likely to commit suicide,
although he may try to self harm, but I don't think there's much chance
of him doing so.' Making inferences from factual information about
the future is becoming an increasingly important part of health care,
for example, in 'risk assessment' and 'assessment of dangerousness'.

The sentence shows that the writer is aware of what might happen in such situations – and so is a 'good' mental health professional in waiting – yet these possibilities are expressed as so unlikely that nothing needs to be done.

It is a common reaction when a nurse is required to present a formal piece of writing to fear the criticism of those who read it. This might be the case, for example, if a nurse is asked to write a case summary on a client for presentation at a multidisciplinary meeting. But such concerns extend to all the written texts a nurse might be involved in, for example daily reports, assessments, care plans and letters. We can imagine that nurses possess their own internal censor, screening out ungrammatical, contentious or self-incriminating information from their writing, with an eye not simply to what their peers and managers might think of their written communication but also on any future legal investigations into the care of clients. In addition, nurses may be aware that their writings go before them, say something about them, and may be received and judged without any qualification from them as to what exactly they meant to communicate. Let loose to an unknown future audience, any writing that nurses acknowledge with their signatures may seem to them like potential evidence against their abilities.

Of course, some nurses may relish the idea of 'publication' and dissemination of their care work, but these will probably be a minority. It is not surprising that given the threat of future embarrassment or loss of face among peers, or even culpability in court on account of written evidence, nurses fight shy of written texts – keeping what they say 'safe' and suitably provisional. Indeed, such a threat is the stuff that keeps nurses verbal, constructing and negotiating meaning from moment to moment in a spontaneous manner. We might see this preference for spoken language as freeing, allowing the nurse to communicate as with clay, refashioning what one has to say before it sets, discarding it if someone sneers or shakes their head, and beginning again with a fresh supply of language. This moulding of clay is not far from the truth if one observes nurses talking their way to an agreement on a topic – the way the hands move, coax, shape, detail or emphasize the verbal meaning. The importance of non-verbal communication is rendered important when patients are unable to communicate fully, as with stroke patients, post-operative patients or people with hearing disabilities. The writing game is not so easy, as it invariably demands a finished article like china rather than the clay it originated from; it should appear sculpted, smoothed, fired in the kiln. This form of communication requires formality, precision, clarity of grammar and semantic coherence.

Clients and patients, men and gentlemen: who is the subject matter of psychiatry?

Returning to what our nursing students produced, let us consider how the students referred to the 'subject' of the video interview. This will indicate something of how they thought about him. After all, there is

Example 1

some debate as to whether it is best to call people who use mental health services patients or clients, with the term 'client' being argued to imply a more equitable relationship. We found a variety of labels attached to our male subject: *man, patient, gentleman, client* and *person*, in descending order of popularity. Each of the 26 students chose one, two or occasionally three labels for the subject. This was a surprising finding because in a professional group we might expect more homogeneity. There is a tension between professional (non-gendered) and lay (gendered) description of personhood and this may reflect the ambiguous status of the relationship between mental health professionals and the people they deal with. After all, if one is considering compulsory hospital admission, the term 'patient' is the easier one for the circumstances – it implies a medical condition for which treatment is both necessary and urgent. For example, 'The depression seems idiopathic and I would recommend the patient for hospitalization.' On the other hand, someone attending a course of psychotherapy might be more easily thought of as a 'client' as this fits in with the ethos of the discipline – 'client-centred therapy' is a term adopted by one of the major approaches here. For example, a student who did not see the subject as needing hospitalization wrote, 'This *client*'s depression is linked to his lack of social support, as he has moved away from his family and therefore has few people with whom he can talk openly about very personal feelings.' The term 'client' is aligned with a view of his condition as being explicable in social terms rather than being some pathological twitch of his brain chemistry. The terms used to describe the 'subject' are thus flexible. This flexibility may well reflect what the nurse, or the health system in general, is trying to do with the patient or client, man or gentleman. Throughout our own text, we use a similarly diverse set of descriptions of the 'subject'. The reasons behind our own choices of such terms as 'patient', 'client', 'person', 'individual' are partly to do with settings or context (hospital versus community; legislated versus negotiated care) and stylistic preferences.

Sets and purposes: transforming distress into manageable categories

In line with what we said earlier about the business of language for specific purposes (Gunnarson, Nordberg and Linell, 1997), we can tell something about the relationship between the language that is used and the clinical work that has to be undertaken. In the body of data from the students we could detect some prevalent semantic sets, that is, groups of words or terms that share a similar theme or meaning.

Participants	*patient, man, gentleman, interviewer, client*
Social status	*life, family, hospital, job, community*
Negative affect	*depressed, depression, down, trapped, low*
Negative action	*end, suicide, harm*
Negative content	*can't, no, lack* (eye contact), *doesn't, little*
Nursing actions	*support, counselling, therapy*

| Positive effects | *help, better, benefit* |
| Cognition | *feels, needs, feeling, cope, coping, felt, know, need, seems* |

This 'setting' of information is an important part of the process of making sense of patients. In particular, the business of making a record is argued by Berg (1995, 1996) to be crucial to the activity of transforming the patient's problems into manageable ones. These semantic sets not only summarize but transform the information students have at their disposal by reassembling it in a specific manner. The students, then, have been involved in the production of a version of events which is manageable in terms of psychiatry's concepts, categories and working routines. For example, concepts and concerns such as *depression* and *suicide*, *counselling* and *therapy*, and, optimistically, *benefit* all sit easily under the rubric of psychiatric care. In this exercise, and in nursing paperwork in general perhaps, the business of writing 'is a crucial feature of this transformation process' since 'it affords the creation of a re-presentation of the patient' (Berg, 1996, p. 505). Fitting the language into a recognizable genre of nursing talk, then, is part of this process of making the ambiguous material of nature into the kind of material that can be understood and possibly treated with some degree of clinical precision.

Duplicating, doubling and adding precision: why do nurses appear to repeat themselves?

A feature of the texts produced by nursing students was that they often used lists of terms, like *low and depressed*, or *family and work*. These types of lists, usually consisting of two parts joined together, are a common feature of language in the world outside health care too. This feature has been of some interest to linguists, who have coined the term 'binomial expressions'. In the student reports, binomial expressions such as *anxious and depressed* appeared to be a significant feature. Binomial expressions have been discussed at some length in legal language by Mellinkoff (1963) and Gustafsson (1984). These authors distinguish two categories of binomials: those that are merely 'worthless doubling' of synonyms (Mellinkoff, 1963, p. 349) and those that are needed for technical accuracy because 'to a lay person the two words mean the same thing, but to members of the [legal] profession there is a clear distinction' (Gustafsson, 1984, p. 134). Thus, in these terms, *low and depressed* might be worthless doubling, whereas *anxious and depressed* or *life and himself* might add to the picture because the words have different meanings.

So far we have been taking a rather strict, dictionary definition approach to the use of multiple terms. In addition, there are a number of social reasons why listed terms might be used. For example, we should note the finding from research on eyewitness testimony that more detailed recollections are more convincing to the hearer (Bell and Loftus, 1988, 1989). Moreover, in producing convincing accounts of unusual or hard-to-believe phenomena, details are often included,

Example 1

possibly as a way of making the teller's account more vivid (Wooffitt, 1992). Thus, perhaps in our data we have the same process at work, insofar as participants are including lists of descriptive terms or alternatives. Therefore, maybe adding terms into the account does important work as a feature of the nursing register. Some of the expressions used by students took the form of clichés like *family and friends* – this is a 'fixed expression' (Moon, 1994) which has general recognition and usage.

A good many of the binomial expressions (those in two parts) related to the feelings of the patient in the video or some judgement on his mental state. That is, the students used paired items like *nervous and very depressed*; *nervous and trapped*; *confidence and courage* and *suicide and self harm*. This is indicative of a strong focus on problems. Moreover, they are predominantly problems that can be located in the individual and described in terms of individual states and properties. This is unsurprising, as English contains a far richer set of terms for describing individuals than it does for situations or places (Allport and Odbert, 1936). Indeed, as Ross (1977) notes, there is a strong tendency for observers to emphasize the role of the person and discount the role of the situation.

Moreover, there is a correspondence between the use of binomial expressions and the assessment and intervention emphasis of the nursing process. In this way the nursing students are producing accounts of the patient which emphasize that his problems are susceptible to intervention. Something, in other words, in which psychiatry should have a stake and which can and should be worked upon.

Assessing the subject's condition: adverbs and the generation of diversity

We were struck by the apparent inconsistency in the way the subject's condition was described in such a variety of ways. This diversity was located primarily in the use of adverbs, that is, words that modify adjectives, verbs or other adverbs and which express manner, degree and circumstance. The adverbs that occurred most frequently in our nursing texts fell into the categories described by Johansson (1993). They were adverbs of degree and extent; emphasis; time; evaluation of truth; and quality and state. The category of degree and extent contains those adverbs linked to diagnostic function (*severely* or *significantly* depressed) and personal appearance (*slightly* untidy, slouched *slightly*). Of particular interest is the discrepancy in the assessment of the patient's physical appearance found elsewhere. One participant described the patient's appearance as *smartly dressed* as opposed to *slightly untidy*. The diagnostic function also features in the category of quality and state (*clinically*). Adverbs of emphasis (*obviously, clearly, particularly, only, simply, really, specifically*) all lend a rhetoric of certainty to the observations. However, adverbs that evaluate truth are duly sceptical about phenomena (*apparently, possibly*). The dominant temporal focus of the texts is upon the recent past (*recently*).

The majority of the students referred to the man as *depressed* (28 occurrences in 26 texts). An examination of the ways that the adjective is modified reveals that where modification occurs there are a number of terms used: *clinically, very, severely, significantly, moderately*. These appear to be used synonymously and without due regard for precise agreement of definition and it is almost as if the diagnosis is being applied in an arbitrary fashion.

So, even though there is a kind of generic consistency to the way students write about the depressed person, there is also a puzzling diversity which can be located largely in the use of adverbs. There are important implications for practice here. This wide variation in the use of modifying terms does not clearly assess the level of depression as exhibited by the person interviewed, although there is some consensus in terms of severity. Thus, they appear to be using a rather loose intuitive yardstick. Given the concerns we have raised elsewhere about 'linguistic entrapment' (Crawford, Nolan and Brown, 1995), it is easy to see how judgements of this kind can be detrimental to patients. One implication for nurse education and practice would be to emphasize to students the need to restrict the use of diagnostic terms like 'depression' to cases where a diagnosis has been established using recognized criteria, rather than use the term indiscriminately. Thus we would advocate that nursing students follow a rubric or set of guidelines for clinical expression. Whereas there are moves to characterize and classify the activities involved in nursing (Clark and Lang, 1992) and encourage more comprehensive documentation (Allen, 1994; Gruber and Gruber, 1990), the problem is that no generally agreed rubric or convention exists for clinical expression in nursing records. As we argue later, we need a balance between a rigid framework for nursing expression on the one hand and a complete lack of one on the other.

The precision of terms used has long been a central concern of many other professions. The legal and scientific disciplines have recognized that the teaching of the definitions implicit in core, technical vocabulary items is necessary for new members of the discipline. Swales (1990, p. 111) says, 'From the way that an economist defines "wealth" or a sociologist defines "class" or a political scientist defines "liberty" we can get an immediate insight into his basic thinking.'

In our texts, students are deploying words that are significant, but are not sufficiently aware of the narrow semantic range of these words, that is the limitations imposed upon the use of such words. When they use the term *clinically depressed* they are not applying the specific diagnostic criteria used in the psychiatric discipline, from the *Diagnostic and Statistical Manual* (American Psychiatric Association, 1994) or the International Classification of Diseases (World Health Organisation, 1992). The term denotes a condition for which treatment is required or which the person is unable to cope with by themselves. Strictly speaking, it should be applied only in response to such defined criteria being met and is therefore not open to free and unrestricted use. This also applied to the term *depressed* as opposed to *low* or *down*.

Example 1

Equally, terms such as *very* or *significantly* are devoid of precise psychiatric meaning and therefore limited in usefulness. Of course, a great deal of psychological vocabulary has entered popular culture over the years: 'People more dejected and unhappy than usual often say they are "depressed". In most cases what they are describing is a perfectly normal mood swing . . . The use of the term confuses a normal mood with a clinical syndrome' (Comer, 1995, p. 270).

The students in this exercise are perhaps accomplishing this transition through their use of clinical terms mixed in with their own adverbs or modifiers. This is an important linguistic sign of a broader social process at work – that of bringing the person's everyday problems into something that they as would-be professionals can have a stake in. This process of repackaging the material as a clinical issue can have negative implications too. As Swales (1990) points out, some words have a rigid, narrow definition, others can be paraphrased, and some are so imprecise that we might even want to redefine them. Freely using linguistic terms such as *clinically depressed* or *depressed*, without having sufficient evidence for using them, can falsely position and indeed potentially incarcerate individuals within medico-nursing records which have lasting effects.

There are two major implications we can draw here. One is to see this as a technical problem in nursing education. Perhaps nursing students need to be provided with clear definitions of technical vocabulary and have impressed upon them the importance of not paraphrasing these terms, and retaining their precise meaning and use. The second implication is more complex and involves seeing the students as altogether more canny or shrewd. In describing the subject as *clinically depressed* they are importing and producing their own precision. Precision does not exist inherently in the interview, so it has to be worked up by splicing this raw material with something more clinical. Accomplishing this leakage from one language style to another may also be seen in the use of lay terms such as *low/down* rather than the precise term *depressed*. Here, the vagueness may be persuasively significant (Potter, 1996, p. 166), as it may facilitate a slippage between everyday unhappiness and psychopathology.

We have highlighted variations that occur in the assessment of the patient with regard to adverbs. The contradictory descriptions of appearance and diagnosis should alert us to the potential damaging consequences of such imprecision.

There are also some important theoretical implications in this tendency of the students to be extremely glib about attributing emotional states and psychopathologies to the patient. Being presented with a person in this context immediately sets up for them an 'explanation slot' (Antaki, 1994) which professionals typically fill with diagnoses, explanations and prognoses. Their use of lay terms like *low* or *down*, their use of modals and their rather hasty diagnostic judgements make up a package that does several things. At its simplest level, it might establish which side of the boundary between depressed and non-depressed the patient falls. However, it also forms for them and for other professionals what Bhabha (1992) calls a 'productive ambivalence' – a way of thinking through the intersection of symptoms, psychiatric interventions and social mechanisms (Fuchs, 1996). What the students write then is a way of filling the theoretical gap between textbook presentations of mental disorders and future nursing activity. It is as if they are able to say, 'Now I know how to go on.' Moreover, we know from other studies of the words used to characterize patients' emotional problems (e.g. Cremnitier *et al.*, 1995) that the diagnostic process involves perceiving connections between sets of terms. French GPs in Cremnitier *et al.*'s study tended to describe and detect depression in terms of insomnia, anxiety and fatigue. Thus our students are not so much diagnosing patients, as establishing 'diagnostic spaces' in which the patient's problems can be both compressed and unfolded.

The significance of this can be developed further when we consider the process of care and what it means. As Hays (1989) argues, 'Care is not only a physiological and psychological undertaking but also a social, political and ethical encounter. The process is often fluid, intuitive and subjective. And it is precisely the uncontrollable aspects, the disorderly, multidimensional nature of the phenomenon that is so elusive to describe' (p. 203). Thus, we would expect the genre or style of nursing language to reflect this.

The diversity, ambiguity and uncertainty in nursing language may have other origins. Written text in nursing emerges in a field that is already contoured by a range of different policies, intentions and

Key reference

ambitions. As Levine (1989, p. 4) puts it, language in nursing is informed by the ambition 'to create nursing diagnoses through shared, real life clinical experiences' and is hampered by a lack of conceptual coherence due to theories of the nursing process 'competing in an intensely political enterprise'. Hence, we would expect the language of nursing to be ambivalent at many levels. Fragments of meaning from many different theoretical orientations may sediment into it. More importantly from our point of view, the tension between highly literate textbook language in medicine, the 'real life clinical experience', and the ineffability of much of what happens anyway may afford this peculiar position midway between oral and literate culture.

Reported speech: the touch of authenticity

Levine's (1989) interest in how nursing emerges from 'shared real life clinical experiences' sets the stage for a further stylistic feature of student's writing. The material in the videotape is not simply paraphrased or glossed; it is reproduced and reported by the students. Reported speech is found in many of the nursing texts. It is not merely reported, but the participants are specifically orientating to the fact that it is reported in a reflexive or self-conscious manner. This appears to serve legitimizing and evaluating purposes. As Caldas-Coulthard (1994, p. 297) notes, reported speech often betrays authorial interference. We find evidence of this interference or bias in the following extracts:

Example 1

> At the beginning of the interview, he said how low he was feeling, and how much he would like to end it all (though not in these words), and therefore came across as being almost suicidal.

> He states he feels trapped and is only existing, not living . . . He states his job was getting him down and that he's 'always been a homely' person. He appears unreactive and expresses that he is unable to 'pull himself up'. He has a very negative view of life and himself.

The first extract includes a high degree of self-consciousness about the reporting process. Unfortunately, this does not preclude interference. We can see that the rewording of the speech in the reporting process is essential to the legitimization of the author's diagnosis and evaluation. In our second extract we can see the importance of the selection process in reported speech. In other words, the author chooses those lexical items that are most important to her evaluation contained in the final sentence.

The observer may conclude that this use of reported speech is an entirely reasonable practice, but what we have to be aware of is how selection may favour some items while discarding others of equal importance in order to justify the decision arrived at, or as Potter (1996, p. 184) notes, 'one realm of entities' is constructed in the description while another is avoided. This justification of a position is part of a range of legitimizing processes in use in medicine and allows the author to manipulate the facts while at the same time appearing to be faithful to the actual words of the patient. This strategy, which is also employed in journalism, enables the author to appear distant or impartial about facts or events. The students are certainly able to participate competently in this rhetoric of reality construction, and are able to anchor their inferences to the text of the encounter between patient and professional.

Text structure: making problems and providing solutions

It is apparent that the nursing reports are structured according to a 'problem/solution sequence' (Winter, 1986, 1994; Hoey, 1994). Winter points out that texts reflect a 'linguistic consensus' whereby the writer conforms to our expectations of structure and sequence (1994, p. 67). We can see this operating strongly in the nursing process, which focuses on assessment, planning, implementation and evaluation. This pattern is so dominant in the conceptual framework of nursing interventions that the participants reverted to the problem/solution sequence despite the task instructions following a solution/problem format, where participants were asked to recommend whether hospitalization was appropriate, note their observations and give reasons for their decision.

As Berg (1996) notes, texts such as records in medicine have a circular relationship with medical work. The structure of the medical encounter often corresponds to the structure of the forms that have to be filled in and the narrative structure of patients' problems. This frequently happens in research, where the questions asked determine the sorts of responses elicited. In understanding the pervasiveness of a particular structure of storytelling we have to understand a great deal more about the narrative structure of care as a whole.

Qualified nurses' texts: some comparisons with the students

We can note several developments in textual performance by comparing the nursing students in our study to nurses who qualified from the same course of training two years previously. The most significant of these developments is the more sceptical approach of the three qualified respondents concerning phenomena and the solution required. Their remarks often concerned the limitations imposed on the evidence as a result of its being video recorded. Their accounts suggest a more sophisticated and sensitive assessment of interview phenomena than that displayed by student nurses. For example, one of the qualified nurses argued that it was 'difficult to judge self care'. Another wrote, 'Normally I would consider eye contact, but the nature of the interview was such that this was impossible to assess.'

The limited information available in the video was met with a reluctance to make concrete diagnoses. It is important to note that this scepticism is at the level of *evidence*. Whereas the student nurses insert modalizing terms, the qualified nurses are much more exact about their uncertainties. At the same time, a good deal of their professional common sense remains intact. For example, the tacit assumption that self-care is something the diagnostician should be concerned about, or that eye contact, if it could be detected, might be a useful index of mood or self-image, is not subject to the same reflexive scrutiny as the videotaped evidence itself. Overall, the emphasis among the graduate nurses was upon either further assessment of the client's mental state prior to hospitalization, or admission to hospital for assessment.

The reports of our students and qualified nurses are, of course, hypothetical. They will not be acted upon in practice. Although they give evidence of some features of the genre of mental health nursing reports, and provide some clues as to how the students might mature linguistically into qualified nurses, we do not know directly from this example how language works in practice. The next two examples will have a somewhat more practical bent as they are taken from the work of practising nurses. Through these examples we will be attempting to look at some further influences on how stories are told in health care contexts, such as the design of forms, the sociocultural frameworks of interpretation, and the medium of communication.

EXAMPLE 2: WRITING RECORDS AND GENDER ISSUES IN ACCOUNTS OF PATIENTS

Let us now move on to our second example of how we tell the story of clients' distress. This time we shall examine the case of nursing

Example 2

records used by a health authority in the West Midlands (UK) for making notes on clients of the mental health services. We shall distinguish a number of aspects of the form of communication here, but for the moment let us note that there may be immediate, *proximal* relationships which afford the nature of the record, and more distant, *distal* factors establishing its qualities. Our findings here, as in our first example, are not only relevant to mental health nursing but also carry implications for all nursing disciplines.

Let us begin by examining a *proximal* feature, namely the nature of the recording form itself. In this case, how the records tell the story of distress is formulated according to the structure of the records. That is, the forms on which people record their observations have titles such as 'Presenting factors on immediate contact', and 'Profile/Assessment', which includes recreational and work activities, meaningful relationships, community resources, drugs currently being taken, known allergies and general health history. Looking at the first page of the form the nurse making the assessment is confronted with headings like these under which she or he has to fill something in. The structure of the record then in part determines the structure of the interviews and assessments conducted with the patient, the kinds of questions asked and the kind of material the nurse writes down. A good deal of it is *medical* material and this helps to position and identify human distress of this kind as something that fits psychiatry into the canon of medicine and perhaps aids the process of packaging people's difficulties so as to accommodate them in this discipline.

The later pages in the notes have a similar quality, in that the structure of the forms corresponds to the structure of care. There are pages where the nurse is encouraged to establish and write down therapeutic goals for the patient to achieve, evaluations of whether they have been accomplished and a section devoted to a plan of care for the patient. This structure reflects the grand modernist ambition that somehow human ills are susceptible to cure or at least amelioration. The records, in other words, are embedded in a belief system that does not see suffering as divine retribution or as something that purifies the soul. Suffering is composed of problems that can be resolved into goals and techniques for achieving them.

The forms themselves are not ready-made objects. They are a product of evolution; nurses, managers, psychiatrists and others have presumably developed them over a period of time on the basis of their everyday working practices. Equally, they will reflect things that are often missed out – putting a heading on a form is sometimes done to remind those who fill it in to include something that might otherwise be omitted. The language in which the form is phrased – goals and plans, for instance – reflects an urge to process and hasten the patient back to some semblance of normality. The form can be read as a sedimentation of accumulated practical wisdom, tacit theories about what happens and what matters. Before it is even touched by the nurse's pen, the form on which records are written is like an empty cell awaiting the prisoner.

What we have said above about nursing records concerns how we tell the story of clients even before we put pen to paper. Let us now look at how they might be filled in. The following discussion is based on two completed records from the same health authority. Both apply to middle-aged people suffering from anxiety and both were written by the same nurse. Yet they also display the creativity of nurses in negotiating their way through the form's categories. Moreover, this creativity is not purely random, but can be interpreted in terms of broader social currents and processes, especially since one record refers to a man and the other refers to a woman. That is, the more *distal* features of ideology and beliefs about gender afford the frameworks of interpretation within which the story of psychiatric encounters are told. The names are changed to protect the participants' anonymity.

In the two nursing records, which we shall identify with the names 'Jane Addison' and 'John Cooper', there are some clear differences in the way these are written up. The ways in which the records focus on the individuals and their relationships invite comment. Jane's presenting factors on immediate contact are: 'Social factors – pressure at work, . . . [and] possible loss of home and stress leading to anxiety and depression'. So immediately we're presented with a number of aspects that are implied as causal, and that relate to the relationship between the individual and others. John, on the other hand, receives a very different entry in the same place on the form, which asserts: 'Anxiety . . . Agoraphobia – loss of confidence in ability to walk after a recent fall. Loneliness. Physical symptoms of anxiety . . .'. This is more orientated towards establishing therapeutic terms for his distress. The heading 'social' on the form has resulted in some more differences in how the author of the record describes them. That is, Jane's entry reads 'Sees son and his wife regularly . . .' whereas John is described as a 'pleasant genial man . . .'. So John is accounted for in terms of individual characteristics and Jane in terms of relational characteristics. Yet both these individuals are described as suffering from some variant of 'anxiety'. It may be, of course, that this differing interpretation reflects the different ways in which the individuals present their difficulties, and it is difficult to make inference based on two cases. However, the pattern here bears out the suspicion by many feminist scholars that women are seen in terms of relationships more than men. This recollects the way Jenny Kitzinger (1993) analyses the self-help and therapeutic literature that deals with the aftermath of child sex abuse. She locates in this literature an assumption that the women who have undergone this trauma should be aiming to resume heterosexual relationships and sexual activity when their recovery is complete. In other words, women's state of 'health' or 'illness' is conceptualized in terms of their relationships with others.

This is a theme that some feminist critics of the mental health system have identified (e.g. Russell, 1995; Chessler, 1972). That is, if women are culturally supposed to be competent in interpersonal relations and overly reactive to stress, Jane's distress is both a

Example 3

psychological deficiency and an exaggeration of a stereotypical feminine tendency. John's problems on the other hand look like a
technical malfunction, which, because it is nameable, is separable
from his being a 'pleasant, genial man'. Shotter's (1993) ideas about
'social accountability', as discussed in chapter 2, are relevant here.
The complexity of patients' feelings and expressions about their
problems are formulated into goals and the subsequent activity is
collapsed into concerns as to whether these goals are achieved. This
rationality on the part of those who complete the records is accountable – that is, it fits in a justifiable way into the forms of rationality
enshrined in education for nurses and fits with the institutional
practices of mental health care.

Of course, we would not recommend anyone to make substantive
inferences based on just two cases. What we have tried to argue,
however, with the cases of Jane and John is that, even in something
so simple and commonplace as a few remarks about a middle-aged
person with anxiety, there is a whole range of ways in which the record
makes sense as a document that tells you about institutions, gender
and social relationships. The door is wide open for further research
along these lines across all the nursing disciplines.

EXAMPLE 3: HOW WE TELL: THE MEDIUM OF EXPRESSION

A further important aspect of 'how we tell' concerns the medium of
expression. We have already highlighted some of the differences
between speech and writing and indicated why nurses might often
prefer the spoken over the written form. In a sense, written expression
means leaving a hostage to fortune in that someone might criticize it.
Language that is spoken vanishes quickly and gives us the opportunity
to revise, seek feedback and re-explain ourselves. Let us explore these
differences between written and spoken text a little more fully.

Imagine then, the following scenario: a nurse is required to introduce a new structure of nursing care. At first, she thinks that the topic
could be introduced verbally, addressing individual members of her
team and answering any questions and concerns. This informal approach appears a suitable way of informing her team about the
proposed structure and gaining feedback. However, the nurse must
also aim to incorporate the new structure within the hospital's opera-
tional policy – this being a written document which may be examined
by statutory bodies or organizations. Written text demands different
grammar, vocabulary and composition from the spoken language
(Brown and Yule, 1983). Thus, with a certain amount of trepidation,
she sets about the task of writing down the structure, anticipating
criticism from her team – for it is often the case in hospital environments that written policies, regulations or procedures drive a wedge
between management and clinical practice.

Key reference

Let us examine in turn both the nurse's written and spoken
representation of the new nursing structure: the written text having

been the first introduction of the topic to team members – the spoken text being a retrospective between the nurse and one of her team, clarifying the structure's usefulness. By doing this we can establish some of the advantages and limitations of both mediums and take a closer look at what specific differences are evident in each text (the spoken text being transcribed from a tape recording).

Written communication

A NEW NURSING STRUCTURE
It is suggested that:
Nurses work in pairs with a *joint caseload* – thus forming
a *micro-team*. It is hoped that this will: a) maintain
continuity of care (should a member of the micro-team   5
be absent / on leave, then the remaining member will be
knowledgeable of those patients on the joint caseload,
and their respective care plans). b) maximise exchange
of ideas, strategies of care. c) allow for constant feedback, appraisal and encouragement between its members   10
(each nurse no longer feeling isolated, keeping to his/her
individual caseload). d) potentiate mutual responsibility and
shared satisfaction of achievements.

At first glance the above text has a formal outlay – setting out the topic in a structured, point-by-point way. The indication is that the writing has been revised or edited rather than spontaneously created, using a rich vocabulary which reflects the management-style concerns of strategies, feedback and achievements, and terms often used in the nursing profession such as 'caseload', 'continuity', 'care plans', 'appraisal' and 'responsibility'. New terms, which might be emphasized in spoken language by intonation or rhythm, are here italicized. Furthermore, where information is given to clarify a statement, this is established by use of brackets.

This 'relatively fixed, permanent product', as Montgomery (1986, p. 112) calls written text, has been constructed in what experts in grammar would call a subject-predicate form. The subject – the new nursing structure which is specified in the first four lines – is followed, after the colon in line 4, by the predicate, which in this case involves the listing of points a, b, c, d. Thus, the text assumes a concise or concentrated form, and chopped syntax (grammatical arrangement of words) in which listed points refer back to the subject in order to complete the sense of what is written. Line spacing is utilized to separate information in a logical manner: the title from the introductory clause, and that in turn from the paragraphed proposals. For all these reasons the text presupposes the 'process of interpretation' of written language as something that may be 'extended, deferred and interrupted', involving several readings and re-readings (Montgomery, 1986, p. 112).

The tone of the written text, although formal and documentary, does include clauses that try to package the proposals in a less definite,

Example 3

subjective manner, e.g. 'It is suggested', 'It is hoped'. Such compromises highlight an intention to strike a balance with the reader – the nurse – trying to soften the blow of a formal, alienating document. As Brown and Yule (1983, p. 5) suggest, 'The writer has no access to immediate feedback and simply has to imagine the reader's reaction.'

Whereas, in spoken language, pause, intonation, pace, rhythm and paralinguistic behaviour (e.g. facial expressions and gestures) demarcate what is said, written language has to rely heavily on syntax, punctuation, capitalization, italicization, paragraphing, etc. In the above text, for example, dynamic action words such as 'maximise' (line 8) and 'potentiate' (line 12) come at the head of each deferred clause, thereby stamping or emphasizing what follows. The notion of 'caseload', central to the new nursing structure, is emphasized by repetition within the text. In addition, the logical connector 'thus' (line 3) substitutes for less formal development of ideas in speech.

All in all, taking into consideration the general context in which the above text was constructed, both advantages and disadvantages for choosing such a medium are apparent. It serves, as Jack Goody (1977) suggests, two functions in particular. It has a 'storage function, that permits communication over time and space' and it 'shifts language from the aural to the visual domain – permitting examination outside of its original contexts' (Goody, 1977, p. 78).

The written text allows the reader to read and re-read, to reflect on what is proposed, backtracking if needs be, deciphering its meaning. However, the written text does not permit a flexible and exploratory introduction of the topic. This transactional, rather than interactional, nature of written text concurs with Stubbs (1980, p. 100): 'Many of the differences in form, particularly in grammar, between spoken and written language are due to the different purposes they serve, and are especially due to the rather restricted and specialized functions of most written language.' It is precisely a specialized function (the need to have a permanent text) which necessitated the topic of joint caseloads and the setting up of micro-teams being encapsulated in writing.

Spoken communication

Transcription from a recorded conversation

A: erm ++ basically I'm I'm not too sure whether + people understand + what I'm going on about as regards erm the micro-team ++ have you any ideas ? +++

B: what I think you mean is rather + than + have lots of ++ erm + well + there's a team of two nurses + working closely together ++

A: erm ++ my idea is that if you have two working together + yeah ? you're going to + have + basically you're going to have better continuity of care (B: mmm) yeah ? (mmhum) + am I wrong ?

B: no you're right (A: all right) ++

A: and + also + you're going to feel less like + you know + a lone ranger + erm or something like that +++

B: think it's good + to be able to discuss + a patient with someone who knows what's going on ++

Disregarding the problems of transcription we have here, as Ong (1982) puts it – in a style befitting David Attenborough – the word in its 'natural [oral] habitat' (p. 8) has many characteristics and qualities not shared by the written medium. Let us look at some of these.

This dynamic, interactive, though transcribed conversation in a face-to-face setting shows an 'instantaneous and collaborative engagement' (Montgomery, 1986, p. 112) which is impossible in written text. Imagining, as we have to in this case, a whole host of conceptual phenomena and paralinguistic behaviour, we can see both A and B discussing in an exploratory, informal manner the topic, moulding as if with clay the object of meaning. This process has distinctive features.

Firstly, the spoken text has pauses (indicated by +) which do not correspond in distribution to punctuation in writing. Sometimes these occur roughly at the boundaries of a sentence or clause (e.g. 'there's a team of two nurses +') but this is not always the case ('and + also +'). These pauses may be seen to derive from the problem of planning speech while simultaneously producing it, and as indicators that a 'turn of talk' is over ('have you any ideas ? + + +').

Often, in place of or in conjunction with pauses, the spoken text has 'erms' or fillers, vocalized in a level tone to distinguish them from say the checking 'eh?' which has rising intonation. Thus potential or actual gaps in the flow of speech are filled, indicating the current turn of talk is to be continued.

Vital to any spoken discourse is back-channel behaviour. This verbal or non-verbal phenomenon is the way that the non-speaking participant shows reactions or alignment to what is said. The non-verbal aspect is not evident in the transcribed text, but we can see verbal examples that fail to support ('mmm') and support ('mmhum') what the speaker is saying.

Furthermore, it is symptomatic of the informal, exploratory nature of spoken discourse that markers of sympathetic circularity (Brown and Yule, 1983) are used, inviting the listener to assume the speaker's point of view (e.g. 'you know'). This degree of verbal imprecision or inexplicitness, reflected also by the use of generalized vocabulary like 'lots of' and 'something like that', serves the purpose of the discourse that is trying to escape formality, trying to build a framework of shared understanding.

Within this less dense network of incomplete sentences and clauses in spoken discourse, where there is the constraint of having to make up what is said spontaneously, repetition of words ('basically I'm'), ideas ('two nurses working together') and syntax ('you're going to') occurs. We are also likely to find false starts whereby an utterance is left unfinished and replaced by something else, as in: 'have lots of + + erm + well + there's a team of two nurses'.

We can see, then, that speech has the sort of flexibility that writing invariably lacks. This suits its use as a means of shared communication

Example 3

of an informal and co-constructive nature. Of the many advantages this medium allows, one stands out in relation to the task of promoting the new nursing structure: the potential for discovering or uncovering meaning without the obstacle of formality and the possibility of alienating peers who may resent a procedural, written text. However, because of the transitory nature of speech, this medium would not suffice for the need to communicate over time and space. Where in the written text a nurse may backtrack and view once more a written text, thus aiding remembrance and consolidation, this proves difficult with spoken discourse.

We may say that, in the context of introducing the new nursing structure, both speech and writing were equally useful. Each with its own intrinsic logic and value, they allowed, respectively, for communication over time and space and for sufficient shared understanding. A written text, in isolation, without subsequent verbal discussion may have alienated those reading it. Yet, spoken discourse alone would not have brought the clarity and permanence of ideas into play. As with pottery, much of nursing language, be it spoken or written, offers the opportunity to mould and discard in order to begin again, and the opportunity to mould and keep.

A large part of language performance involves persuasion. Persuasive language is important if we as nurses are going to get our point across, or in advertising parlance, sell ourselves or our ideas. In the case of spoken language we can see that there is a persuasive element where the new structure is sold as a way of solving problems in nursing. The actions of the nurse informing others about the desirability of the new structure can be seen as a kind of 'interressement' – 'by which an entity attempts to impose or stabilize the identity of other actors it defines, through its problematisation' (Callon, 1986, pp. 207–8). That is, one actor says something about the identities of other actors. You have an identity (you are a nurse) yet you are hampered in achieving valuable parts of that identity (ensuring continuity of care, being able to discuss patients with trusted colleagues), but by using the new structure these problems can be avoided.

This resembles advertisements that identify a problem, like children touching things with germs on, and promote a product such as a spray-on disinfectant to avoid this. At the core of such persuasion is one's identity as a good parent – or, particularly, mother – and one's inevitable concern to keep one's children away from germs. In our example we can see the nurse promoting this new mode of working as an 'entity' who is trying to enrol other 'entities' such as other nurses, and more broadly the institution, its core values and even the patients into this new structure. This kind of persuasion is achieved by interposing oneself and one's ideas between the targets of one's persuasion – other nurses – and presenting the new ideas as a pathway that improves the relationship between the target entity and his or her core professional values (Michael, 1997).

THE IMPLICATIONS OF LANGUAGE STUDY: FROM THE TRAINING OF NURSES TO CONCEPTIONS OF HEALTH CARE

The implications of what we have written so far should be understood in the context of a growing belief that nursing language should be addressed more comprehensively in the training of nurses, and bear on the question of whether nurses are indeed firing paper bullets at patients or merely letting off blanks. Our conclusions are broadly of two types. Firstly, we can make suggestions for the practice of nursing and nurse education. That is, our examples suggest that relevant nursing bodies need to develop the curriculum further to include language awareness. There is a need for textual management in nursing informed by an awareness of both positive and negative aspects of report making.

Secondly, we can draw some conclusions of a more conceptual kind which bear on the study of language in health care contexts. Under this heading we would draw attention to our findings concerning the marked linguistic features of psychiatric nursing reports. In the first part of the chapter, about the texts produced by the nursing students, we noted the high incidence of lexical items such as *feel* and *need* compared to texts in general. Such items could be read as reflecting humanistic or client-centred concerns and contrast with the more distant and scientific style one expects from medical discourse. At the same time, it could reflect what Miller and Rose (1994) call an 'orthopaedics of the soul' whereby therapeutic theory and practice subject the client to a kind of authority or regulation. Talking about a client in terms of feelings and needs then might serve a regulatory function as it unfolds the spaces into which the client's distress can then be packaged.

With Jane and John too, we can see this packaging process at work. The form of communication, or how we tell stories about human distress and suffering, is unfolded along lines laid out in the structure of recording forms, the structure of health care systems and the social and cultural currents that afford the spaces into which disability and distress can intelligibly unfold.

With spoken and written communication we can also see how the form and function of language are conditioned by what people are doing with it. The feedback, mutuality and collaborative construction of the spoken version help to enrol other nurses into agreement with the new structure.

A finding in the reports produced by students with both practical and conceptual implications concerns the frequent use of modality terms. This suggests that the participants are unable or unwilling to write definitively. Opinions are given in a such a way as to invalidate their worth by heavy use of modalities, such as *seems* and *appears*. The participants are unsure about what conclusions to draw based on what they have seen. These 'intermediate modalities' are opposed to 'categorical modalities', which Fairclough (1989) argues support 'a view of the world as transparent – as if it signalled its own meaning to any observer, without the need for interpretation and representation' (p. 129). In fact, we might argue that uncertainty is not all bad and indeed might be offering a kind of resistance or buffer to the more categorical and empowered style of medical language. Future investigation might seek to explore whether this moderation of illocutionary force does indeed 'say nothing' as Levine (1989) feared it might. On the other hand there may be good reasons why reports about patients take this form.

In addition to the use of modal terms, another area of uncertainty involves the variation between different nurses' accounts. The wide adverbial variation in the assessment of the subject's condition is surely a matter of practical concern. This might be expected concerning the diagnosis, but was even more remarkable for the patient's physical appearance. After all, on the basis of the reports we can have at one extreme a *smartly dressed, moderately depressed* person, and at the other a *slightly untidy, severely depressed* person. As such we have two different subjects, not one. If we account for all descriptive permutations, we extend the 'fragmentation of the subject' further. Perhaps some effort in training nurses so that their observations converge would be desirable. In many other disciplines based on observation and description, such as botany, a good deal of effort is put in to ensure that students describe specimens in a way that corresponds to the established standards of the field. It is surely all the more important that human beings are granted the same descriptive consistency as botanical specimens. This does not necessarily mean that descriptions correspond with reality, but it does ensure consistent community of understanding among the observers.

The diversity in participants' descriptions even extended to a marked heterogeneity in the labelling of the subject in our first example by both student and graduate nurses. These, as we have seen, ranged from *man* to *gentleman*, and *patient* to *client*. One graduate nurse countered distance and anonymity by using a fictional but personal name 'Tom'. Such variety suggests that the participants are lacking in consensus about the status of those who need psychiatric care. The low use of the term *client* may well correspond to its ambivalent status in health care. The term tends to be associated with reformist rhetorics of user empowerment. These form an uneasy bridge between traditional medical model orientations and more radical, politicized concerns to prioritize the interests of the user. Perhaps this heterogeneity corresponds to the currently fragmented nature of the philosophy of mental health care. Again, it is interesting to speculate as to whether or not this diversity might be reduced if there were a greater commonalty in the 'ways of seeing' (Berger, 1972) encouraged by trainings for nurses.

On the other hand there is some evidence for a cohesive philosophy of care if we look differently at the words used. The prevalent 'semantic sets' we identified highlight a strong structural and topical 'cohesion' (Halliday and Hasan, 1976) to the reports that focus on the patient's cognition, emotion, motivation, social status, negative factors or deficits, and the benefits of nursing interventions. This cohesion is part of the problem/solution text structure identified by Winter (1986, 1994) and Hoey (1994). The wide use of reported speech in the reports again add to our sense of these reports as manufactured on a language production line, within tight generic rules. This concern with speech and dialogue in nursing language might be one of the points of leverage to shift us to a more dialogical rather than monological style, a feature that seems suited to its mission of communicating with fellow professionals and fits with the oral culture of nursing. The conversational style of nursing language has been noted elsewhere (Fisher, 1995) and may offer opportunities for reform to make health care more democratic. We can only welcome a fuller communication as nurses enter the lifeworlds (Mishler, 1984) of clients.

In our analysis of how nursing students used reported speech from the client we warned of the dangers of taking this technique for granted and of not paying attention to the ideological functions of selectivity. In writing about clients, both in our exercise for students and in nursing records as a whole, nurses do not note the analytic work that goes into these everyday judgements. Like the 'common sense' we described in chapter 2 there is an automatic quality to the way in which clients are packaged into the reports and records. There was some acknowledgement of the provisional or incomplete status of the data on the part of the graduate nurses. However, they were no more sceptical in making their observations and recommendations. The process of getting the job done, filling in the form, or implementing whatever is flavour of the month in terms of nursing management strategy meticulously disengages the critical faculties of the nurse. It is relatively rare for nurses to stop in mid-task to ask 'Why are we doing this?'

Perhaps if they did it would be a good thing. The few minutes lost in reflection would be amply repaid in terms of the insight gained. We would argue that reflexivity or self-consciousness is a valuable analytical skill for nurses. Attending to the basis on which we make our judgements and communicate with others might give some insight into why discrepancies have arisen and why communication and care look the way they do in institutional contexts. If we accept the view that social reality is a human construction, examining language gives us some clues as to how people are – often unconsciously – going about arranging it. Whether the 'loaded weapon' (Bolinger, 1980) of language is used to fire paper bullets or mere blanks, the mechanism must be understood.

This chapter has begun to describe and to analyse aspects of 'how we tell' in nursing language and to raise awareness about the difficulties, traps or limitations that such language can have. Apart from adding to knowledge about the linguistic features of nursing reports, our study has exposed their uncertain and at times conflicting nature. On occasions contradictory details of the patient emerged, as did different styles of contextualizing male and female patients, and the style of communication varied dramatically depending on whether it was spoken or written.

The business of transforming the unruly world of health care life into written language presents nurses with a problem similar to that of journalists telling stories about reality. Like the journalist, nurses 'begin with predefined notions about the form of their report, which in turn leads them to shape the content of the message' (Altheide and Snow, 1979, p. 62; Bing and Lombardo, 1997).

In dealing with these forms, genres and conventions of description, nurses should become more aware of the power of language. Nurses need to become as cautious and attentive to language as they are to changes in blood pressure or body temperature. Language is not a sideshow. It is where power is embedded, in the forms, genres and conventions of expression, and where, as Fairclough (1989) notes, the struggle for social emancipation can take place. Reform of language so as to avoid any abuse of power against those in our care can only begin by first describing and then analysing that language. Critical linguistics provides some framework for establishing critical reading of subject positions and classification and can help guard against naïve communication or maintaining an imbalance of power in speech and writing. Yet such an approach must be backed by a willingness on the part of educators to build on these findings by bringing language issues into the nursing curriculum. There needs to be a language component in training curricula, tailored specifically to already widely established concerns regarding the generation of meanings in texts. This suggests that some improvement can be made in the degree to which students can be helped to acquire a technical register that equates with a standard of professionalism but does not incarcerate those for whom they care in future.

So, finally, how does nursing language exert power and reveal its own power relations? We have not answered this question here, but we have begun our answer by describing and analysing features of nursing language. We have raised the alarm that nurses might be firing potentially damaging 'paper bullets' at their patients, without even knowing that they are doing it. On the other hand, nurses may be 'firing blanks' in the sense that they do not state their position or viewpoint authoritatively and use language forms that meticulously avoid certainty.

CONCLUSIONS

There is something distinctive about the language of nursing. Its form is detectable through studies of word frequency, styles of expression, text structure and even the structure of records. The desire to assist patients and relieve suffering which is at the heart of nursing values is best achieved, we would argue, by a constant vigilance about nursing language. Nurses need to choose between merely regurgitating the categories and assumptions soaked up in their training or genuinely tailoring their use of language to what the patient might benefit from. They need to question whether they are fitting the patient to the form or more properly fitting the form to the patient. The distrust of paperwork, memoranda and forms which many nurses feel, surely reflects the way that written text, in conceptual and linguistic terms, is a million miles from what nurses do, say and think when they are at work with patients.

We have not offered, nor do we intend to offer, any formal, detailed guidelines as to what nurses should do to avoid 'linguistically entrapping' patients. Certainly, as yet it is unlikely that preceptors, mentors or even professors of nursing are sufficiently aware of the problematic issues surrounding the language of nursing dealt with in this book. However, we do not wish to make nurses feel hopelessly guilty about firing paper bullets at patients. By raising awareness of the difficulties and problems inherent in nursing language, we hope to make nurses better placed to challenge and question not just their own language acts but also those of other individuals and groups involved in health care. We do not offer an easily digestible model of language practice which nurses can apply like Roper, Logan and Tierney's (1985) activities of daily living. There is not that kind of comfort zone here. Instead, we hope to inspire a *deeper* concern and scepticism about language so that nurses can begin to resist *in their own way*, in ways yet undefined, language acts that are detrimental to the people they care for.

SUMMARY

We have used three kinds of examples to argue that there is a distinctive form to nursing language. Firstly, word frequencies and styles of expression were examined in reports from mental health nursing students commenting on a videotaped interview with a depressed man. This suggested a distinctive use of pronouns, terms and modal forms which characterizes the genre of mental health nursing. Also noted were tendencies to express the condition of the person in the video in rather florid terms like 'severely depressed', 'moderately depressed' or even with the stamp of medical authority, 'clinically depressed'. We have examined how the student nurses used these terms, and have emphasized the need for them to be aware of the precise meanings these have in psychiatry as distinct from lay language and to be aware also of the implications their language has for the patient. Language is closely allied with the course of action the students wished to take with this subject and the attempts they wanted to make to alleviate his condition. Without careful scrutiny of the injudicious use of language these therapeutic manoeuvres might just as easily lead to him being trapped rather than helped.

The second example attempted to show how the way patients are written about and hence thought of is influenced by the features of the setting within which and for which the writing is done. Even the design of forms, we have argued, has a bearing on the kinds of information that are recorded. Moreover, the form of the story we tell may be aligned with and informed by broader cultural values and ideas. In our case there was a correspondence between the way our two patients were written about and broader ideas about women and men.

Our third example explored the relationship between spoken and written text, where these were argued to be distinctive by virtue of their different choice of words and structure and the immediacy of feedback from an audience in spoken communication.

Thus we have outlined how the texts found in nursing have a distinctive flavour, shape and form. It is by developing awareness of this that we may enable caring work to assist clients and guard against the possibility of nursing language trapping them.

REFERENCES

Allen, A. (1994) Does your documentation defend or discredit? *Journal of Post Anaesthesia Nursing*, 9(3) 172–3.

Allport, G.W. and Odbert, H.S. (1936) Trait names: a psycho-lexical study. *Psychological Monographs, Basic and Applied*, 47(211).

American Psychiatric Association (1994) *Diagnostic and Statistical Manual of Mental Disorders*, 4th edn (DSMIV), American Psychiatric Association, Washington.

Antaki, C. (1994) *Explaining and Arguing*, Sage, London and Thousand Oaks, CA.

Altheide, D.L. and Snow, R.P. (1979) *Media Logic*, Sage, Beverley Hills, CA.

Bell, B.E. and Loftus, E. (1988) Degree of detail of eyewitness testimony and mock juror judgements. *Journal of Applied Social Psychology*, 18, 1171–92.

Bell, B.E. and Loftus, E. (1989) Trivial persuasion in the courtroom: the power of (a few) minor details. *Journal of Personality and Social Psychology*, 56, 669–79.

Berg, M. (1995) Turning a practice into a science: reconceptualising post-war medical practice. *Social Studies of Science*, 25, 436–76.

Berg, M. (1996) Practices of reading and writing: the constitutive role of the patient record in medical work. *Sociology of Health and Illness*, 18(4), 499–524.

Berger, J. (1972) *Ways of Seeing*, Penguin, Harmondsworth.

Bhabha, H.K. (1992) The other question: the stereotype and colonial discourse, in *The Sexual Subject: A Screen Reader* (ed. M. Merck), Routledge, London and New York.

Bing, J.M. and Lombardo, L.X. (1997) Talking past each other about sexual harassment: an exploration of frames for understanding. *Discourse and Society*, 8(3), 293–311.

Boden, D. (1994) *The Business of Talk: Organisations in Action*, Polity Press, Cambridge.

Bolinger, D. (1980) *Language: The Loaded Weapon*, Longman, London.

Caldas-Coulthard, C.R. (1994) On reporting reporting: the representation of speech in factual and fictional narratives, in *Advances in Written Text Analysis* (ed. M. Coulthard), Routledge, London, pp. 295–308.

Callon, M. (1986) Some elements in a sociology of translation: domestication of the scallops and fishermen of St. Brieuc Bay, in *Power, Action and Belief* (ed. J. Law), Routledge & Kegan Paul, London.

Cheek, J. and Rudge, T. (1994) Nursing as a textually mediated reality. *Nursing Inquiry*, 1, 15–22.

Chessler, P. (1972) *Women and Madness*, Doubleday, New York.

Clark, J. and Lang, N. (1992) Nursing's next advance: nn internal classification for nursing practice. *International Nursing Review*, 39(4), 109–12.

Comer, R. (1995) *Abnormal Psychology*, 2nd edn, W.H. Freeman, New York.

Crawford, P., Nolan, P. and Brown, B. (1995) Linguistic entrapment: medico-nursing biographies as fictions. *Journal of Advanced Nursing*, 22, 1141–8.

Cremnitier, D., Guelfi, J.D., Fourestie, V. and Fermanian, J. (1995) Analysis of the terms used by general practitioners to characterise patients considered by them to be depressed: a prospective study of 682 patients. *Journal of Affective Disorders*, 34, 311–18.

Encandela, J.A. (1991) Danger at sea: social hierarchy and social solidarity. *Journal of Contemporary Ethnography*, 20(2), 131–56.

Fairclough, N. (1989) *Language and Power*, Longman, London.

Fisher, S. (1995) *Nursing Wounds: Nurse Practitioners, Doctors, Women Patients and the Negotiation of Meaning*, Rutgers University Press, New Brunswick, NJ.

Fuchs, C.J. (1996) Michael Jackson's penis, in *Cruising the Performative* (eds S.E. Case, P. Brett and S.L. Foster), Indiana University Press, Bloomington.

Garfinkel, H. (1967) *Studies in Ethnomethodology*, Prentice Hall, Englewood Cliffs, NJ.

Giglioni, P.P. (1972, Ed.) *Language and Social Context*, Penguin, Harmondsworth.

Goody, J. (1977) *The Domestication of the Savage Mind*, Cambridge University Press, Cambridge.

Gruber, M. and Gruber, J.M. (1990) Nursing malpractice: the importance of documentation or saved by the pen! *Gastroenterology Nursing*, 12(4), 255–9.

Gunnarson, B.L., Nordberg, B. and Linell, P. (1997) *The Construction of Professional Discourse*, Addison Wesley Longman, Harlow, UK.

Gustafsson, M. (1984) The syntactic features of binomial expressions in legal English. *Text*, 4(1–3), 123–41.

Halliday, M.A.K. and Hasan, R. (1976) *Cohesion in English*, Longman, London.

Hays, J.C. (1989) Voices in the record. *Image: Journal of Nursing Scholarship*, 21(4), 200–3.

Hoey, M. (1994) Signalling in discourse: a functional analysis of a common pattern in written and spoken English, in *Advances in Written Text Analysis* (ed. M. Coulthard), Routledge, London, pp. 26–45.

Johanssen, S. (1993) 'Sweetly oblivious': Some aspects of adverb–adjective combinations in present-day English. In *Data, Description, Discourse: Papers on the English Language in Honour of John Sinclair* (ed. M. Hoey), HarperCollins, London.

Kitzinger, J. (1993) Sexual violence and compulsory heterosexuality. In *Heterosexuality: A Feminism and Psychology Reader* (eds S. Wilkinson and C. Kitzinger) Sage Publications Inc., London.

Lakoff, R. (1975) *Language and Women's Place*, Harper & Row, New York.

Latour, B. and Woolgar, S. (1986) *Laboratory Life: The Construction of Scientific Facts*, 2nd edn, Princeton University Press, Princeton, NJ.

Martin, J.R. (1984) Language, register and genre. In *Children Writing: A Reader* (ed. J.R. Martin) Deakin University Press, Geelong, Victoria.

Mellinkoff, D. (1963) *The Language of the Law*, Little Brown, London.

Michael, M. (1997) Individualistic humans: social constructionism, identity and change. *Theory and Psychology*, 7(3), 311–36.

Miller, P. and Rose, N. (1994) On therapeutic authority: psychoanalytical expertise under advanced liberalism. *History of the Human Sciences*, 7(3), 29–64.

Mishler, E.G. (1984) *The Discourse of Medicine: Dialectics of Medical Interviews*, Ablex, Norwood, NJ.

Montgomery, M. (1986) *An Introduction to Language and Society*, Routledge & Kegan Paul, London.

Moon, R. (1994) The analysis of fixed expressions in text, in *Advances in Written Text Analysis* (ed. M. Coulthard), Routledge, London.

Ong, W.J. (1982) *Orality and Literacy: The Technologizing of the Word*, Methuen, London.

Potter, J. and Wetherell, M. (1987) *Discourse and Social Psychology: Beyond Attitudes and Behaviour*, Sage, London and Beverley Hills, CA.

Proctor, A., Morse, J.M. and Khonsari, E.S. (1996) Sounds of comfort in the trauma center: how nurses talk to patients in pain. *Social Science and Medicine*, **42**(12), 1669–80.

Psathas, G. (1995) *Conversation Analysis: The Study of Talk in Interaction*, Sage, London.

Romero, C., (1986) The grisly truth about facts, in *Reading the News* (eds R.K. Manoff and M. Schudson), Pantheon, New York.

Roper, N., Logan, W. and Tierney, A. (1985) *The Elements of Nursing*, Churchill Livingstone, Edinburgh.

Ross, L.D. (1977) The intuitive psychologist and his shortcomings: distortions in the attribution process, in *Advances in Experimental Social Psychology*, vol. 10 (ed. L. Berkowitz), Academic Press, New York.

Russell, D. (1995) *Women, Madness and Medicine*, Polity, Cambridge.

Shotter, J. (1993) *Conversational Realities: Constructing Life Through Language*, Sage Publications Inc., London.

Shotter, J. (1997) Review of Fisher, S. *Nursing Wounds*, New Brunswick, NJ: Rutgers University Press. *Discourse and Society*, 8(1), 154–5.

Stubbs, M. (1980) *Language and Literacy: The Sociolinguistics of Reading and Writing*, Routledge & Kegan Paul, London.

Swales, J.M. (1990) *Genre Analysis: English in Academic and Research Settings*, Cambridge University Press, Cambridge.

Winter, E.O. (1986) Clause relations as information structure: two basic text structures in English, in *Talking about Text* (ed. M. Coulthard), Birmingham University, Birmingham, pp. 88–108.

Winter, E.O. (1994) Clause relations as information structure: two basic text structures in English. In *Advances in Written Text Analysis* (ed. M. Coulthard), Routledge, London.

Wodak, R. (1996) *Disorders of Discourse*, Addison Wesley Longman, Harlow, UK.

Wooffitt, R. (1992) *Telling Tales of the Unexpected*, Harvester Wheatsheaf, Brighton.

World Health Organisation (1992) *The ICD-10 Classification of Mental and Behavioural Disorders: Cultural Descriptions and Diagnostic Guidelines*, World Health Organisation, Geneva.

KEY REFERENCES

Brown, G. and Yule, G. (1983) *Discourse Analysis*, Cambridge University Press, Cambridge.

Hewitt, J.P. and Stokes, R. (1975) Disclaimers. *American Sociological Review*, 40, 1–11.

Levine, M.E. (1989) The ethics of nursing rhetoric. *Image: The Journal of Nursing Scholarship*, 21(1), 4–6.

Potter, J. (1996) *Representing Reality*, Sage, London.

4 MEANING: WHAT DO WE TELL?

AIMS

This chapter aims to establish how difficult it is to define meaning and how it is best understood in the context of culture and social action in health care.

Nurses should gain an appreciation of the contributions of semiology (the study of signs) and hermeneutics (the art or science of interpretation) to the study of meaning, and how authors in sociology, feminism and cultural studies have developed and transformed these ideas so as to think about how meaning works and circulates within societies as a whole.

We shall show how meanings exist because communities of people work together to create them and how the response of the hearers is as important as the intentions of the speakers in fixing the meaning of communication and enlisting clients' agreement in diagnosing the problem. This should lead to an appreciation of the construction of meaning by health care professionals and how patients ascribe meanings to their problems.

The chapter should enable nurses to become more aware of the communication style of their encounters and the records they construct about patients. We aim to create suspicion that, even when there is an emphasis on clients' own narratives, needs, wants and desires, there may still be a process of medical management at work which mutes the client's voice or perspective. Finally, we wish to re-emphasize that meaning is a disorderly, multidimensional, jointly produced phenomenon.

INTRODUCTION: WHAT IS MEANING? DEFINITIONS AND EXAMPLES

We have all asked the question 'What do you mean?' or 'What does that mean?' Sometimes we have asked ourselves the question 'What do I mean when I say that?' Nurses frequently come up against the uncertain meaning of the words people use. Meaning is often difficult to pin down. What might patients *mean* when they complain of 'pain', 'depression' or 'feeling lousy'? What do they *mean* when they say, 'I'm feeling much better?' Do they *mean* they feel physically better or mentally better? Are they feeling 'better' about one or several aspects of their lives? Are they saying this in order to convince themselves that they are better and ready to be discharged? Are they saying this to make others more comfortable around them, when really there has been no change or even a deterioration in their health? The search for the meaning *behind* words can seem like unpacking boxes to see what is concealed in them. But what exactly do we find? What exactly is meaning? The problem of defining meaning has puzzled linguists and philosophers for centuries, and has never been satisfactorily resolved. There is no generally agreed definition of meaning. Picking up a dictionary, we might see meaning defined in terms of intention, purpose, result, reference, indication or as definition itself. However, looking at meaning in everyday life in care settings is not advanced much by this. Perhaps we need a more ethnographic understanding of meaning, such as that provided by Dahlgren (1988, p. 287): 'By meaning I refer here to the processes of making sense of the world around us. It has to do with creating a general coherence in our lives.'

As we are concerned with a realm of activity in health care, we might wish to draw on the philosopher Wittgenstein's edict, 'the meaning is the use'. This would direct us to examine the meaning of terms by looking at how they are used in health care. As Wittgenstein put it, 'Try not to think of understanding as a mental process at all . . . but ask yourself: in what sort of case . . . do we say, "Now I know how to go on." In other words, one's aim is the practical one of enlarging (and transforming) one's current reality to incorporate a text's message, its subjective strangeness being rendered familiar in the process.' (Quoted in Shotter, 1983, p. 270.)

This implies that the meaning of something can be understood in terms of the subsequent intentions or actions of a person for whom that thing has meaning. A further elaboration of this position can be seen in Coulter's (1979) argument that a thing is meaningful if it achieves some sort of public criteria or recognition. For example, in a study of health and illness in a small rural community in Mexico, Castro (1995, p. 1013) notes how villagers would sometimes account for the death of someone as being caused by pain: 'They say he died of pain,' as one informant said. In the UK or USA it is not common to see pain itself as lethal. As we saw in chapter 2, Castro's informants also used the same words – gordo or gorda – to refer to being healthy and being plump or fat. In poor parts of the world this makes sense, as putting on weight can be taken as a sign that one is doing well; rather than, for example, in Europe and the USA, where excess weight is seen as a risk factor for illness and as aesthetically unappealing. So to make sense of what health and disease mean, we need to explore the values, ideas and circumstances of the community as a whole, within whose context health and disease are experienced.

Key reference

Different cultures, then, may use different symbols of health and disease and communicate about them differently. The interchange or exchange of meaningful symbols has been central also to a number of theoretical currents and schools in social psychology. The influential historian and social psychologist Rom Harre promotes 'the idea that social interaction is mediated by public performances which are treated by social actors as signs. They are operative through their meanings, that is conventional associations, and not through causal powers as physical objects in the world' (Harre, 1979, p. 63).

In this case, the meaning of a thing is defined in terms of its effect on the subsequent meaningful action (or 'praxis') by other actors. Meaning is a social phenomenon in this view, and is both produced and conventionalized. We draw on conventions, norms, rules and common sense to manufacture meaning in our daily lives.

MEANING, CULTURE AND SOCIAL ACTION

Whatever meaning is, then, it is rich in culture and social action. One of the paradoxes of what meaning involves is that it is easy and difficult at the same time. It is relatively easy for socially competent people to say what something means, yet it is extremely difficult to provide a watertight definition of meaning which would withstand scrutiny by social scientists or philosophers. Meaning is 'content rich' in that it is difficult to examine without reference to something specific that is meaningful. Consequently, in the remainder of this chapter we will work through a series of examples of how meaning has been conceptualized and deployed in health care encounters.

An extension of the strand of thinking which assigns a social role to meaning is opened up to us if we begin to understand the anthropological perspectives that may be raised on the healing process. Even modern scientific medicine, psychiatry and therapy come uncannily close to Deborah Glik's (1990) description of healing in other cultures and in alternative medicines: 'The promise of healings of bodily mental and spiritual ills is of central importance to understand the attraction of persons to groups that practice ritual healing' (p. 151). In a similar vein Kleinman, working in Taiwan, documented how healing assisted people in coping with a variety of disease, distress or unfavourable personal circumstances (Kleinman, 1980). The meaning, in this view, that people attach to the illness or the circumstances that face them is vitally important in making sense of what they do.

Key reference

In Glik's (1990) study of people seeking spiritual healing experiences in the USA she noted that they often presented with rather diffuse problems and experienced healing that effectively redefined their problems. The more willing they were to redefine their problems the more healing they claimed to have experienced. This often took place within a stream of thinking where both mundane and extraordinary events are given a sacred meaning. Amongst the cases Glik describes, there was a young man who was dissatisfied with his lack of education and his low-paying job as a 'gas station attendant'. During the study he was cured of warts and skin problems and pain that he had suffered from since being in a car accident. His major presenting problem, the lack of opportunity or education, was unresolved, yet his redefinition of the situation enabled him to feel that the healing process had been successful. As some of Glik's respondents said, ' "God works in mysterious ways", a popular phrase among the participants who typically believe that the seeker of healing should not be too specific about what is to be healed' (p. 163). Meaning in this context is something that is deployed flexibly and in line with changing circumstances. The meaning of having been cured is attached to the changes that occur. Indeed one's preparedness to be this flexible is a good sign at the outset of the healing process.

Let us, perhaps rather fancifully, extend this analogy of healing in other countries and contexts a little further. The officially recognized, textbook-sanctioned basis of Euro-American medicine, the physiology of the individual, is only part of the story. Any new way of telling the story of healing in modern medical contexts must grapple with the social and linguistic dimensions. Let us, then, consider hospitals as factories for packaging distress in ways that can be dealt with and about which a meaningful story can be told. From the man who is troubled by the spirit of his dead grandfather to the person whose increasing mobility difficulties render her a suitable candidate for hip replacement, the health system formulates the problems in living in such a way that they can be administered, costed, managed and in some cases treated.

CLASSICAL TRADITIONS: SEMIOTICS AND HERMENEUTICS

In order to get a grip on what is meant by meaning, we shall take a brief digression through two traditions that have contributed greatly to the academic debate on meaning in language and text whose relevance to nursing, we hope, will become clear. What we shall describe are two traditions that originated in the late nineteenth and early twentieth centuries, namely semiology (or as the Americans say, following Peirce, semiotics), and hermeneutics. Both of these arose in relation to the puzzle over how it is that human signs, languages and texts have meaning.

Early this century Ferdinand de Saussure originated semiology or the study of signs (see Saussure, 1974). He was keen to search for the stable, structural features of all languages and this led him to focus on the distinction between the *signifier*, which is the signal or sound pattern of language, and the *signified*, which is the concept or meaning attached to that signal or sound pattern. This is based on the commonplace observation that we might say 'chair' in English but 'chaise' in French. The signifier may differ but what is signified or signalled in both cases is the meaning element of the chair. The chair that is signified is an abstract one. The signified 'chair' exists in the collective consciousness of the English-speaking community, and the signified 'chaise' exists in the collective consciousness of the French-speaking community. It is important to remember that the signified is a concept and does not correspond to any particular concrete object.

Saussure, and subsequent thinkers like Peirce (1935–66) and Barthes (1967) have adhered to this sharp split between the sign (signifier) and its meaning (signified). By means of sign systems 'reality' is created. This view came to be called 'structuralism'. This view holds that in any given culture language *structures* reality; it decides, if you like, what you do, say, think or experience. As the twentieth century wore on, a variety of scholars attempted to explore the structure of symbol systems and human social life. Linguists such as Edward Sapir (1921) and Benjamin Lee Whorf (1956) took these ideas in a strong form to argue that language organized and determined thought and perception. Anthropologists such as Claude Levi-Strauss (1963) examined how the structure of social life was bound up with the way non-western societies named objects, spoke to each other and undertook kinship relations, while Roland Barthes (1973) followed up the Saussurean emphasis by examining signs and myths in contemporary cultures.

The psychoanalyst Jacques Lacan (1977a, 1977b) theorized that the unconscious is structured by language and that it is through language that the child comes to acquire the ability to distinguish between self and other. In his view, the symbolic order has historically been dominated by men and so is masculine or 'phallic'. Louis Althusser (e.g. 1968, 1969) examined the constructed nature of reality in relation to a Marxist understanding of the power of ideology. Ideology operates as a superior structure to language in a particular community and works to constrain the possible meanings of a sign within that community. Althusser is associated with the view that ideology 'interpellates' human subjects; that is, it makes possible or controls our lives and even our understanding of ourselves as subjects.

This picture of our being unable to resist the power of sign systems and ideologies as they interpellate our subjectivity and mould our thinking is increasingly challenged by feminist critics who see language as rich in opportunities for resistance too. Julia Kristeva (1984; Moi, 1986) identifies a realm of language and sense making – *la semiotique* – which underlies, yet is autonomous from, Lacan's phallocentric 'symbolic order'. Helene Cixous (e.g. 1981; Probyn, 1993) began to unpick the masculine or phallocentric focus of Lacan's interpretation of Freud. The linguistic, speaking subject, in her view, is always gendered and embedded in power hierarchies. Traditionally, in health care settings doctors have predominantly been men and, since the nineteenth century at least, nurses have been women. The nurse, then, speaks in an often hostile enunciative ground when talking to her medical colleagues – little wonder that nurses are often hesitant and tremulous in offering opinions or questioning medical expertise. As Stuart Hall (1990) has added, 'Practices of representation always implicate the positions from which we speak or write – the positions of enunciation . . . though we speak, so to say, in our own name, of ourselves and from our own experience, nevertheless, who speaks, and the subject who is spoken of are never identical, never in exactly the same place' (p. 222).

This gendered positioning that goes into language has prompted Luce Irigaray (1985) to begin to describe a style of writing she calls 'ecriture feminine' which subverts the dominance or hegemony of male imaginations and enables women to escape from the silence patriarchy imposes on them. We shall return to these points in the final chapter, which is concerned with how we might tell stories in health care differently. For the moment let us note that, according to these authors, ideologies and structures of language are important in determining forms of thought and the kinds of people we can be.

There are, however, loopholes constructed within feminine language which escape the iron grip of patriarchal ideology.

Let us go back for a moment to Saussure's division between *signifier* and *signified*, which is far trickier than first appears. Opposed to those who we might call 'structuralists' are 'poststructuralists' who persistently problematize the meanings, that is, the signifieds and concepts of signs, images and words. This critique of straightforward correspondence between signs and their meanings is perhaps rather commonsensical. After all, when people say 'cow' they do not always mean a 'female of any bovine animal'; they might, for example mean a 'highly objectionable person or thing'; or an 'ugly or bad-tempered woman' (courtesy of *The Penguin English Dictionary*). A reduced, simple image of a suitcase at a railway station may 'stand for' the place you find baggage; but a realistic image of a suitcase without such a context may 'stand as' a suitcase. The linguistic sign, as Saussure indicates, is arbitrary because it can be replaced with something else. Thus if we agree to call a 'table' a 'dog' then we will all sit down and eat our dinner at the dog! Or we may say, 'Lay the dog for dinner'! Furthermore, meanings of words change over time, or from one place to another, or between different readers. In effect words do not simply mean something. Ambiguity, of course, is not always clear on first inspection. Certain signifiers might seem unproblematic, such as 'up' or 'down'. It appears easily within common sense to know the meaning of the signs 'up' and 'down'. But even these can be problematical. What about if 'up' and 'down' concern mood states rather than spatial position? Words and combinations of words often have multiple meanings. What appears to constrain them, or straitjacket them if you like, is the context in which they occur.

The context in which words or signs appear affects the range of meanings we derive from them. We can say that such and such a sign means this in a certain context. So that when we ask for dinner to be put out on the table, an interpretation of 'table' as an item of furniture may safely be arrived at. Or the meaning of saying 'He's going to jump' may refer to several different kinds of 'jumping' actions, yet we would not think of an athletics meeting when these words are delivered on an acute psychiatric ward. Context may include the words that surround a word, or its collocations. Thus, we might comfortably distinguish what 'rose' means in the context of 'watering can' and what it means in relation to 'bread'. Many of the signs (spoken, written, visual) that we use are highly abstract. For example, how many meanings might we give to 'soul' or 'spirit'? Other difficulties can arise when words with quite different meanings have the same pronunciation or sound – something which often leads to humorous confusion. Furthermore, different cultures can place quite different meanings on everyday words. To the young Afro-Caribbean population, for example, 'bad' might mean 'good'. Homosexual activists might proudly reclaim derogatory terms like 'queer' (Smythe, 1992) or 'dyke'. 'Sick' is a state of the body, the act of vomiting, or a way of saying we disapprove of something. Meaning only loosely and ambiguously attaches to collectivities of words. To understand meaning we have also to understand collectivities of people. Although context often channels meaning, the meanings of many of the words and combinations of words that we use are not so easily constrained by it. Here lies great difficulty. We have to rely on interpretations that are not always, and perhaps can never be, completely accurate.

A huge amount of communication in nursing is what we may think of as being 'loose' in meaning. This 'looseness' or generality makes for speedy, easy and often thoughtless communication. For example, a nurse might say, 'Watch out for Bill – he can be very difficult.' We might substitute several alternatives for 'difficult' – 'dangerous', 'childish', 'irritable', 'nervous', 'manipulative', 'unpredictable'. The looseness of meaning serves laziness and avoids tighter analysis and assessment. Sadly such comments as 'Watch out for Bill – he can be very difficult' are accepted at face value and form the baseline for observing 'Bill' and fitting his behaviour to suit the comment. For example, a nurse might meet Bill and think, 'He isn't speaking very much. Yes, Bill is very difficult – he doesn't speak.' Perhaps, the argument we would make here is that, if nurses are going to make general comments that encourage wild or free interpretation, they should, where possible, make positive ones such as, 'You'll like Bill – he's easy to get on with.' Such a statement might lead a fellow nurse to think, 'He isn't speaking very much. Yes, he is very nice – very easy to work with. Although he doesn't say a lot.'

The complication to the question of meaning has been magnified by the work of Jacques Derrida (1976, 1978), where the problem of words not having core meanings at all is powerfully emphasized. Derrida breaks with those who believe words refer to things. He shows that words refer to other words which again refer to others and so on without end. This also applies to texts as a whole. Texts refer to other texts and so on – a phenomenon we referred to earlier as 'intertextuality'. This inability to *mean* in any thoroughgoing way has posed difficult questions for those concerned with the meaning of language. Such a view of signs as not merely arbitrary in nature but incapable of having meaning in any total way has had a dizzying effect on our experience of spoken and written text. We wonder whether anything that is said or written can be truly interpreted or whether it is subject to endless possible interpretations. Derrida, and those who have followed him, such as Geoffrey Hartman (1980, 1981), J. Hillis Miller (1982, 1992) and Paul de Man (1979, 1984, 1986), have indicated that texts do not have an authoritative voice that points to a 'truth' beyond words. Texts are riddled with rhetoric, and, when they are challenged or critiqued to show contradictions and ambiguity, lose their authority. Thus 'meaning' is deconstructed or broken down. Other theorists such as Stanley Fish (1972, 1980), Hans Robert Jauss (1982) and Wolfgang Iser (1974, 1978) introduced the perspective of the reader and the way texts are received. This reader-response criticism brings into play the view that readers construct the texts they read and fill in the gaps in meaning that all texts have with the fruit of their own lived experience and past reading.

So far we have been dealing with words and with styles of speaking and representation. Once words have been composed into texts the problem of what they mean multiplies even further. The interpretation of texts, especially the Bible, has been subject to a great deal of debate and it is from this approach that our second major interpretive tradition, hermeneutics, emerges.

Interpretation or hermeneutics has had a lively history in biblical study, where issues arise about differences between versions of the text and the problem of translation from original biblical languages such as Hebrew, Aramaic and Greek, and Latin translations of these, into mainstream, living or vernacular languages such as English or Spanish. We might ask whether we can ever arrive, for example, at the original words of Jesus Christ, the so called *ipsissima verba* or actual words, through the various sieves of editing and translation. These are questions for biblical scholarship, of course, but what they do illustrate is that texts and words do not simply travel down the generations with fixed meanings.

Texts and the words that make up those texts are constantly subject to new and at times contradictory interpretations. The problem of making sense of the Bible is arguably comparable to the problem of making sense of people in the human sciences. Hermeneutics is concerned to make the most defensible reading of a relatively obscure text (Ricouer, 1971). One cannot prove that any particular interpretation is correct, merely that it is the most defensible. As Ricouer argues, hermeneutics is thus rather like a complex case in a court of law. Which of several different accounts is the most persuasive or the most likely? As Hudson (1984) reminds us, the ambiguity in interpreting texts, be they accounts of patients' symptoms or hastily scribbled patient records, might open up recesses of experience which more formal methods of enquiry might fail to reach. The diversity of interpretations which hermeneutics, properly applied, might raise is an asset rather than a problem.

SOCIAL MEANINGS, INTERACTIVE MEANINGS

The meaning-making process in health care is a social one. Making sense of what is going on as a nurse or as a researcher involves being able to make sense of this sociability. We are in many cases dealing with a community of healers and the sick, who share beliefs about what happens and what matters in the healing process. In studies of literature and the media, scholars have come up with the notion of an 'interpretive community' to characterize the situation.

Thomas Lindlof writes a densely argued justification for the concept of the 'interpretive community', as an account of how meaning comes to be held in common:

> . . . the existence of agreement on a conceptual category indicates
> a high frequency of communication on the subject, exposure to the
> same types of verbal and non-verbal performance, and enactment

> in roughly similar . . . situations for the persons that are sampled. From the socially constructed meaning approach, then, consensus does not advance the warrant for an objectified reality . . . A full accounting of such agreements as they are revealed in socially co-ordinated practice would result in a cultural level of explanation that is not reducible to primitive psychological or physiological terms. This is the level at which an interpretive community concept can be proposed.
>
> *(Lindlof, 1988, p. 87)*

Thus, if a number of people in a health care setting, for example, agree on what it is that is happening – that they are removing someone's appendix or administering supportive psychotherapy – then as social scientists we should be looking at how this agreement is accomplished by means of their social practices. The organic condition of the patient alone does not tell us exactly how healers will consider it, talk about it or attempt to treat it.

The shared meaning of the human condition and the borrowings between different theoretical schools of health care was illustrated for one of the authors (BB). A friend became increasingly distressed about how her career as an optician seemed to be blocked by her superiors at work and she was not getting on well with her family. She consulted a homeopathic practitioner, whose solution was to provide her with a pill. Sure enough, the situation at work and among her family began, in her view, to improve. Now, even the most optimistic neuropharmacologist in conventional psychiatry could not provide a detailed account in chemical terms of how tablets could lead to career advancement or more satisfying family relationships. Yet it is hard to make sense of this healing practice without seeing both the practitioner and the patient as borrowing from the signals, symbols and ceremonies of conventional medicine. Administering pills for human ills has a specific history, and becomes accountable as a sensible thing to do with distress because we have grown up in a world that views the human body and the human social milieu as something that can be regulated, supervised and enhanced chemically. Whether by means of conventional or homeopathic models of chemistry, we can see that both draw on similar tacit models of health and disease which enable patients and practitioners to participate as healers and the healed.

In this context it is important to note how Duck (1994) emphasizes the importance of sharing meaning in social relationships, 'by which I mean the deep processes of understanding someone else's ways of thinking about their experience in the world' (p. xv). The common structures of meaning between different situations yield the means by which people can participate in social life. Meanings, in our sense, then, are things that are created between people. Meanings depend on the speaker and the hearer. The social theorist and philosopher George Herbert Mead had this to say: 'The act or adjustive response of the second organism gives to the gesture of the first organism the meaning that it has' (Mead, 1967, p. 78). The hearer's response to the speaker constructs the meaning of the response for both partners (Shotter, 1987). We will say more on this in chapter 5 on 'audience'.

To examine this possibility a little more fully, perhaps it is worth considering what patients themselves have said and done about the care they have received. Overall, many people who receive care will say that it is adequate or even helpful. On the face of it, the meaning of clinical interventions is fairly clear. Yes, people do find them effective. In study after study, across a whole range of human ills, treatment groups outperform control groups, as they live longer, experience less pain or report themselves to be less depressed, depending on what it was that brought them into a health care setting in the first place. Indeed, if the cumulative improvements in health reported in the literature were added together we would all live to be happy, pain-free 100-year-olds. Clearly, though, life isn't like that. Why not exactly?

CONVERSATIONS AND NEGOTIATIONS IN ESTABLISHING CLINICAL MEANING

Perhaps one place to look for an answer is in the way meaning is negotiated in clinical settings. Maybe one reason why clinical work is not so clear-cut is that the sufferer and the clinicians have some latitude to work out what is wrong, what counts as treatment and what counts as an improvement. Indeed, this might be especially true once we move away from the often carefully selected participants in research studies, who represent ideal types of the various syndromes treated, and look at the rather less clearly defined troubles of everyday life.

Analysts such as Douglas Maynard have documented the work that goes on in clinical encounters to set up the problem and subsequent course of action. To give you an idea of what this involves, let us consider the example of medical encounters in a study by Maynard (1991) of talk in clinics that specialize in childhood disorders like autism and developmental disabilities. Children were assessed and then clinicians met the parents to discuss the nature of the child's problems and provide recommendations for therapies and treatments and advice on dealing with specific difficulties. As clinicians introduce their findings and recommendations to the parents, they often ask parents for their perspective on the child and incorporate this into their report. At first glance one can see how this works, in that it is often difficult to tell people that their child has a problem, so aligning their diagnosis with the parents' tale of woe makes it more palatable. Maynard called these encounters perspective display series (PDS), which involve: (1) the clinician's opinion, query or perspective display invitation; (2) the recipient's reply or assessment; and (3) the clinician's report and assessment. Clinicians tend to fit their diagnostic news delivery to the occasioned display of the parents' perspective, especially by formulating agreement in such a way as to co-implicate the parents' perspective in the diagnostic presentation. The clinician's invitation (phase (1) above) could be marked or unmarked. Marked invitations look something like the example that follows, and involve a formulation of the problem as somehow being possessed by the child.

(14.012 simplified and adapted)

Dr E: What do you think is his problem?
Dr E: I think you know him better than all of us really. So that you know this really has to be in some ways a team effort to understand what's going on.
Mrs D: Well I know he has a learning problem in general and speech problem and a language problem [and] a behaviour problem. I know he has all of that, but still at the back of my mind I feel that he's to some degree retarded.

(Maynard, 1991, p. 168)

These are 'marked' invitations because the clinician says the child has a problem. The clinician's question is 'presumptive' in that it contains a suggestion or proposal that requires acceptance. An 'unmarked' invitation does not propose a problem. Here is an example:

(9.001 simplified and adapted)

Dr S: Now that you've – we've been through all this I just wanted to know from you how you see J at this time.
Mrs C: The same.
Dr S: Which is?
Mrs C: Uhm, she can't talk.

(Maynard, 1991, p. 172)

This begins with a rather more open-ended invitation by the clinician and does not presume so much about the child. However it also smoothes the route to delivery of diagnostic news. If problems are identified and described by the parents, then the diagnosis looks more confirmatory than presumptive, and allows our imaginary clinician to say something like 'Well, this is what we've found too, and the medical name for this is . . .' Thus, by establishing the alignment of language, clinicians can establish agreement as to what the problem is and what possible treatment or therapy options might be. Let us consider another example which involves the refusal of a marked invitation by the parent:

(22.007 simplified and adapted)

Dr N: It's obvious that you understand a fair amount about what Charles' problem is.
Mrs G: Yeh.
Dr N: So at this point there is a certain amount of confusion.
Mrs G: Mm hmm.
Dr N: In your mind probably as to what the problem really is?
Mrs G: Mm.

Dr N: And we haven't really had a chance to hear from you at
          all as to what you feel about the situation.
Mrs G: Well I don't think there's anything wrong with him.

(Maynard, 1991, p. 173)

This sequence is rather more drawn out and the clinician has to make
a number of gambits to get a response other than 'Mm' out of the
hearer. This tendency to disagree hesitantly in conversation is common
when people wish to demur from the 'preference structure' (Pomerantz, 1984). We will return to the business of patients – and their
parents – refusing or modifying diagnostic news later. For the moment,
the important feature is the conversational gambits that participants
use to create jointly the meaning of what is wrong.

Marked and unmarked invitations differ in terms of what follows
in the sequence. Marked invitations are 'suggestions or proposals that
require acceptance'. If parents disagree that the problem resides in the
child the interactive work of modifying that disagreement has to be
accomplished and the parents' positions modified in ways that sustain
the clinician's claim to expertise. The unmarked invitation's alignment
between parents' and clinicians' views is sought but in a different way.
It enables parents to provide indications that something is wrong
which the clinician can then elaborate on so that their diagnoses
appear more confirmatory than presumptive. As Maynard (1991)
writes, 'A result of strategically employing these various procedures
. . . is to maximize the potential for presenting clinical assessments as
agreeing with recipient's perspectives or in a publicly affirmative and
non-conflicting manner' (p. 87). So, formulating the meaning of
symptoms, pains or difficulties in living is a somewhat disorderly joint
process, complete with false starts, disagreements and hesitations.
Language is the glue we use to attach the fragments together so as to
establish a system of meaning which has its own coherence and
consistency.

FROM THE MEANING OF CONVERSATIONS TO THE MEANING OF LIFE

Moreover, through the achievement of agreement between the participants, we can see how they are able to align themselves with the
'grand narratives of their social world' (McAdams, 1993, p. 265). In   **Key reference**
everyday conversation, we often say that someone has 'found meaning
in their life' in the sense of becoming happy, fully functional, adjusted,
free of anxiety and so forth. Although conversation analysts like
Maynard try to avoid making forays 'under the skull' to explain social
behaviour, it is tempting to see how clinicians can presumably align
themselves with identities, roles or values that give meaning to their
work. Being a healer, bringing relief where there is suffering or
knowledge where there is confusion, may figure as part of this.
Although all this is highly speculative, there are ways of making sense
of the processes involved. Perhaps, as McAdams (1993) suggests, there

are a variety of resources of meaning we can draw on to make sense of our lives.

McAdams describes his own theory of how we ascribe meanings to ourselves and our activities, using what he calls *imagoes*. An imago is like a role, for example the nurse role, doctor role or patient role, but in McAdam's formulation there is a good deal more to it – the imago involves the values attached to the role too. They are like idealized characters in myths or like ancient Greek gods, who each had a specific domain of responsibility. In modern-day personal meanings, McAdams identifies imagoes such as 'the healer', 'the teacher' or 'the counsellor'. Whereas this might seem fanciful, one can see some correspondence between the ideas here and professional values and ethics that pervade everyday practice. Just look at what it means to describe someone as 'unprofessional' – it is usually part of a major and fundamental criticism, and is often part of the charges at disciplinary hearings. The business of core professional values – the imago of the healer, if you will – is often called upon in discussing controversial issues in medicine. For example, at what stage should life support machines be turned off, or under what circumstances should people be treated against their will? The answers to these questions are often referred back to values such as the reduction of suffering or the prevention of greater harm at a later date. Meaning, and particularly the meaning of one's work in health care, is central in negotiating professional identities and stories in the workplace of health care.

A further complication to this picture emerges in terms of how staff cope with their values, stories or imagoes being frustrated. Patients may fail to get well, be unappreciative or even commit suicide. Here the resilience of staff may be taxed severely. For example, a friend of one of the authors (BB) who was working in liaison psychiatry related how a client had made two suicide attempts, the second one successful. Here, her point of view was almost one of heroism in the face of futility; being a good psychiatric nurse is about facing such challenges – rather reminiscent of the poem which begins 'If you can keep your head when all about you are losing theirs . . .'. The virtue, then, in this healer's imago is its very robustness, that it cannot be thwarted or set back despite the suffering in the world.

There is another effect of these imagoes or professional life stories. From our point of view, one of their important effects is to individualize health care. Coping with work, or with clients who die of overdoses, is seen as a problem that the professional on his or her own has to confront. There is little room in this professional life-storying for an account of society, where there are profound social inequalities in health – where indicators as diverse as mortality, morbidity, incidence of tuberculosis, birth weight and children's' height offer a far less favourable picture in situations of poverty and social deprivation (Eames, Ben-Shlomo and Marmot, 1993; Reading, Raybould and Jarvis 1993; Spence *et al.*, 1993; Townsend, Phillmore and Beattie, 1988). In an editorial in the *British Medical Journal* in 1993, Smith and Eggar made an impassioned plea for policy makers, researchers and medical staff to take more notice of the well-demonstrated link between poverty and poorer health. This is more urgent, they argue, than looking at diet, smoking and exercise habits. The wealthier classes lived longer too at times in history when it was they who ate more fat, smoked more, took less exercise and more drugs.

Therefore, the meaning nurses assign to their work has important political consequences too. Images of the self as fearlessly tending the sick may not equip them for changing the circumstances in society which produce that sickness or, in the UK, for the growing dominance of managerialist concerns in health care. Indeed, they contribute to encapsulating the meaning of illness as an individuated phenomenon susceptible to individuated solutions. Appeals to professionalism, to the image of fearless nurses tending the sick out of a sense of duty or love of one's fellow human beings can easily be used to deflect industrial action or to get them to cope with reduced resources.

THE MEANING OF PATIENTHOOD

From the patient's point of view, the meaning assigned to illness has also been a focus of research. For example, Taylor (1989) examined women's stories about breast cancer. Even having undergone surgery, many of the women she interviewed were developing positive meanings from their experience. The search for meaning was aligned with trying to gain a feeling of self-mastery over the events in order to manage them. Hence we can make sense of the women's tendency to attribute the cancer to stress, hereditary factors, poor diet or even, in the case of one woman, to a blow from a flying frisbee. So meanings serve a purpose to the patient.

However, looking at the texture of people's accounts of what being ill is about reveals a somewhat more complex pattern of health and illness in everyday life. Firstly, it is important to note that the experience of illness does not occur in isolation from the rest of everyday life. As Radley (1997) puts it, 'It matters that we are able to do certain things, that we do not let people down, that we go out in spite of our discomforts.' Our everyday behaviour in our bodies 'involves an ongoing accommodation to the smaller or larger perturbations of physical life. It has been shown that people go to the doctor not when their symptoms are at their worst, but when this accommodation to them breaks down (Zola, 1973)' (p. 56).

Key reference

As Radley argues, there may be various means by which this accommodation to the ways of the body becomes sufficiently disrupted to warrant a disease. Here is an account of a man who was diagnosed as having coronary artery disease:

> I was involved in amateur dramatics and we were doing a production. You get tense, even amateurs, before the production, and I started getting the chest pain and at the same time I was worried about redundancy at work and I put it down to just pressures, sort of nervous tension. I was also doing some work for a friend,

> re-wiring his house for him, the pain was getting more frequent and that was about 12 months ago. Then it cleared for a little while and then slowly it came back but not as strong as it had been. I was frightened to work odd times and then I thought 'This chest pain is over-exertion'.
>
> *(Radley, 1988, p. 63)*

So the meanings of changes in one's bodily experience of everyday activity propel one into the medical frame of reference. It is intriguing that this man first accounted for these meanings in terms of his problems and pressures and at this stage it was something he could attend to himself. It was only subsequently that it comes to be made sense of as a condition requiring medical attention. However, there may be circumstances where we resist the bodily problems that beset us, for example, when we keep working to an urgent deadline despite a headache or resist the urge to pass wind or scratch in polite company.

The pathway from being a person to being a patient is complex in psychiatry too. There is a range of factors, described by Goldberg and Huxley (1992), that are involved when someone approaches a general practitioner and in how psychiatric illness is identified by the GP, a referral gets made to a psychiatrist and that referral is dealt with. There are thus a great many filters between the problem first being identified, often by the relatives of the patient rather than patients themselves, and the person becoming a patient.

Rather like Maynard's (1991) example which we quoted above, of parents receiving news about their child's developmental difficulties, there is a drawn-out process of assigning meaning to anomalies in behaviour and bodily sensation. In the end, it is as if professional rhetorics consolidate the somewhat unclear lay notions that something is amiss. The professional packages distress and locates it in some intra-individual way, thus condensing it out of the ill-defined suspicion that something is wrong.

In the case of mental health, Barrett (1991) has shown how the making sense of patients by professionals draws on a variety of registers and modes of speaking. In informal discussions they may draw on lay terminology, describing a patient as 'odd', for example (1991, p. 8). Particularly interesting from our point of view, however, is the way that patients' case records involve a transformation between lay terminology and professional language by means of 'intermediate typifications' – 'words or phrases which bridged "lay" concepts of mental illness and "professional" concepts of schizophrenia' (Barrett, 1991, p. 7). Barrett (1988) has also shown how psychiatrists interviewing patients' relatives frame questions in terms of lay understandings of mental illness. From evidence like this, Parker *et al.* (1995, p. 66) argue that 'Rather than straightforwardly "recognising" psychiatric disorder, professionals could be said to bring forth or construct psychopathology by recourse to a language with which to point to disorder. Thus diagnostic criteria could be said to be justificatory arguments rather than signs.'

This rhetorical field, which has been opened up by writers like Barrett (1991) and Parker *et al.* (1995), who have attempted to scrutinize the linguistic and interpersonal work that goes on in establishing a person's problems, gives us some clues as to the nature of the arguments and disagreements that sometimes go on between patients and professionals.

CONTESTED MEANINGS IN HEALTH CARE: PSYCHIATRY AND CHILDBIRTH

It may be easier to understand the controversial nature of some kinds of health care if we consider its meaning to be ambiguous and up for grabs. This is especially true in psychiatry, where there is some dispute over what people's problems are or what can be done about them. Most textbooks and the majority of psychiatrists and mental nurses see 'mental illness' as somehow roughly comparable to physical illnesses. There is, of course, some measured scepticism about taking the medical model too literally, but the everyday packaging of people's problems draws heavily on vocabularies of 'devastating diseases' and 'illness'. However, there are substantial and often vocal minorities who disagree. The American Psychiatric Association is sometimes beset with demonstrations by ex-patients at its conferences who argue that psychiatry has victimized them or that their treatment has been oppressive, painful and debilitating. Even though the patients of other medical disciplines experience pain and debility, some of which might well be iatrogenic, that is, caused by medical intervention, it is difficult to imagine a conference of surgeons being besieged in the same way. The troubles and disagreements in psychiatry, however, highlight how variable meanings can be and how the consensus between healers and patients can be fragile.

Indeed, the consumers of psychiatry are, more than the consumers of other branches of health care, apt to problematize the meanings given to their condition by the psychiatric profession and society at large. Emerick (1996) estimates that of the self-help groups for people suffering from so-called 'mental health problems' nearly 80 per cent are anti-professional or anti-psychiatry. Moreover, these groups often espouse a variant of the position that psychiatry is a form of social control. Of the minority of groups he located which adopted a pro-psychiatry or pro-medical model stance, some of these had a high degree of input from parents or relatives of sufferers.

As well as illustrating the contested nature of human distress when it comes to psychiatry, this also highlights how the meaning people assign to their problems is related to their position and interests. That is, if you are the parent of someone who suffers from schizophrenia, it might be in your interests to adopt a medical-model or physical-disease understanding of the problem as this absolves you of any guilt for causing the problem and facilitates alignment with psychiatry, where some sort of solution, however imperfect, might be available.

On the other hand, a sufferer who feels the side effects of medication, or feels trapped within an oppressive collaboration between family and psychiatry, might well adopt a more avowedly anti-psychiatry stance.

The arguments between aggrieved patients and professionals are more obvious in psychiatry. However, we can see the process of negotiating illness and pathological identities at work in other disciplines of care. In a study of women's experiences of childbirth, Woollett and Marshall (1997) present a comment from a participant which illustrates this:

> Interviewer: How do you think your pregnancy went?
> Interviewee: It depends. If you take it clinically, medically, it was wonderful. Otherwise it was bloody awful. I complained every day about it. Because I was so well with [my first child] I didn't know one could be so ill when one is pregnant. I just didn't expect it. I was sick for the first four months, then I had pain in the ribs. . . I couldn't eat and I couldn't walk. I couldn't sleep in the end, I just couldn't enjoy myself at all. Clinically it was OK: I didn't have high blood pressure, swollen ankles, anaemia, what else didn't I have . . . But I felt awful. (p. 181)

Thus, this respondent's comments reflect a tension that it often found in talk about childbirth, where there is some controversy as to how far it is, or should be, a medical process. That is, women who talked to Woollett and Marshall oscillated between accounts of their pregnant bodies as needing to be medically managed and accounts of themselves as experiencing normal healthy signs of being pregnant. As in the quote above, there is also a sense in which the medical version of pregnancy and childbirth missed out a lot of this woman's subjective distress. It could not be packaged into the compartments of bodily malfunction which accompany pregnancy, so it slipped below the line of medico-nursing scrutiny.

THE CHANGING MEANINGS OF HEALTH CARE WORK

As well as the possibly contested meaning between patients and nurses, it is important also to consider what the meanings are which enable nurses to conduct their everyday work in health care settings. In a study of midwives, Harvey (1995) noted how they accounted for themselves as now performing more technically detailed work than they did in the past, at the same time attending to patients' needs in a way that was missed by other specialisms: 'Twenty years ago they couldn't do anything apart from deliver babies. But now they've been given responsibility, because they're good at it, of rupturing membranes whenever necessary, applying fetal scalp electrodes' (Harvey, 1995, p. 771). Despite this increasing technical skill and responsibility it was still an important part of the meaning midwives assigned to their work that they attended to 'the little details, the finer points. You're the only one who's going to do that. The doctors aren't going to do that sort of thing. . . . if we don't do it no one else is going to come along and do it. Someone else might come along and give the IV drugs or do some recordings but they're not going to do the basic things, the human things really' (Harvey, 1995, p. 775).

Thus, there is a great deal that goes on at the level of professional meaning making. In this case there is a sense of 'onwards and upwards', as well as an attention to the basic 'human things' which distinguishes midwives from doctors. As we can see, for midwives this is a very positive and self-affirming identity to give meaning to their work and sustain them through the long hours of labour. We could even say that this kind of identity is important in relation to the work midwives do because they emphasize 'experiential knowledge' of the patient based on caring labour (Rose, 1988). This is in contrast to the piecemeal, technical knowledge that other specialists like doctors have, and is something that the midwives seem to value more highly.

Although the meanings attached to nursing work by nurses and patients are multidimensional, there are some facets that are particularly prominent. One aspect of the subjective experience of nursing, or being a patient, is the sense of control we have over the events that happen around us. Among psychologists studying stress, health and disease, there is a broad consensus that a sense of control is important in being able to cope with events (Bootzin, Acocella and Alloy, 1993; Comer, 1995; Davison and Neale, 1994). A sense of control over potentially stressful events is believed not only to increase our likelihood of dealing with them successfully, but to be better for our bodies too. Our sense of control over events and our ability to cope with them has been related to the functioning of the immune system. That is, poor coping suppresses immune functioning whereas good coping enhances it (Kiecolt-Glaser *et al.*, 1987). A sense of control and effective coping may enable people to get better if they do fall ill too (Rodin and Salovey, 1989). Thus, the meanings we assign to events are important in developing our responses to them. This kind of reasoning lies behind stress management programmes which aim to facilitate coping by giving clients strategies and resources – like the ability to relax – that enhance their sense of control over their responses to events (e.g. Meichenbaum, 1975, 1977, 1993).

That is the story within mainstream psychology at least. From the classic study of cognition and emotion by Schacter and Singer (1962) onwards, it has been supposed that the meaning or 'cognitive appraisal' we attach to events will affect the emotions we experience. The theories or stories we apply to ourselves and to others are powerful factors in happiness, sadness, emotions and stresses.

So much for the evidence and theory within psychology. When we look at the slightly more complex world of nurses, doctors and patients we begin to see some anomalies. The issue of control is one such oddity. At first glance we might guess that it is fairly obvious who controls a situation. Moreover, if one person gains control then the others lose it and vice versa. Consider, then, a study by Molleman and van Knippenberg (1995) where they looked at the changes in attitudes and perceptions when a new nursing regime was introduced in a hospital in The Netherlands. The new system, to put it briefly, involved nurses seeing fewer patients so that there was more continuity of care for the patients themselves; they were cared for by a few 'familiar faces' and not by a plethora of different nurses. Immediately before discharge, patients treated under the new system said they experienced more control. This sense of control extended also to junior nurses while head nurses felt that their control had been reduced. However, there was no perception that anyone else, like doctors, had less control. So where does all this new 'control' come from? Is there a slight shuffling of responsibility from head nurses to humble first-year nurses? The problem is that perceptions of control, the meanings we attach to what is done to us, do not necessarily reflect the political context in which we act. The activities of management boards, banks and governments are difficult to detect when you ask nurses and patients about their work.

WHO GENERATES MEANING? INDIVIDUALS, INSTITUTIONS AND SOCIAL DIVISIONS

To look at this question slightly more broadly, it is customary in Europe and the USA to feel a strong sense of self-determination and autonomy. Indeed, there are substantial literatures attesting to the value of an 'internal locus of control' (Rotter, Seerman and Liverant, 1962) or a sense of 'self-efficacy' (Bandura, 1977). The meanings we are encouraged to assign to our lives are intensely personal – 'I wanted to'; 'I thought it would be a good idea.' Yet at the same time, even a cursory glance at the circumstances of our lives leads to very different implications. We speak a language we did not personally design, we live and work in communities and organizations whose policies, rules and even buildings we did not make ourselves, and inhabit political systems whose democratic basis allows only occasional chances for a change of government. So how autonomous are we? According to many writers, the way we talk is bound up with these structures of power and privilege (e.g. Fairclough, 1989; Ng and Bradac, 1993; Parker, 1992). Indeed, as many have argued, the practice of medicine in the form of psychiatry brings into particularly sharp focus the inequalities in power between those who do the labelling, diagnosis and treatment and their patients (Foucault, 1965; Parker *et al.*, 1995). Health care institutions operate as power structures independently of the intentions of power holders. The effects of hospitals and nursing may be far from what the individual actors intend (Miller and Rose, 1986).

This larger-scale social context of meanings is also informed by the kinds of inequalities that become built into language and regimes of therapy. As an example, take rational emotive therapy (RET), a popular form of psychotherapy originated by Albert Ellis (1962, 1976, 1991). In this kind of psychotherapy the therapist tries to challenge the irrational assumptions in clients' thinking which allegedly underlie depression and anxiety. This is a somewhat directive form of therapy, and in some formulations it can involve some rather sinister techniques and approaches. For example, we can clearly see the operation of social class stereotypes in Young's (1988) account of how this therapy may be done with 'lower class' (*sic*) clients. Young (pp. 80–3) suggests that therapists assume a 'position of command' with such clients, whose attention and respect is most easily gained by using a 'loud voice' or by being touched in a 'forceful, determined way'. In such cases, Young also admonishes therapists to 'establish and exploit a reputation', that is, belabour the point that you are an expert, once again in 'a firm, loud, self-assured voice', and show 'superior wisdom and knowledge'. This is a characterization that should alert us to the problems faced by working-class people or those with little formal education when faced by a therapist. The (presumably unintended) effect of these practices is to consolidate the existing inequalities between therapist and client. Indeed, they bear an unfortunate similarity to the techniques used in the education system by teachers, which deflect working-class pupils away from the more academic streams of work (Willis, 1977). Language, then, can be seen to consolidate class inequalities.

We need to be alert to the possibility that this oppressive and inequitable approach might find its way into the more familiar territory of 'patient education'. Nurses have ample opportunity to slip into the role of expert teacher when educating patients. This powerful and authoritative position over patients may lead to the kind of abuse we discussed above with RET. Health education could be seen as locating the problem within the ignorance of the patient; it is because of not knowing that they become ill. Empowering people through education is about empowering the professional, who in turn confirms the power of professional knowledge.

A more striking example of how meanings are ascribed to language by patients and doctors comes from a case reported in the *British Medical Journal* by Smith (1993) of Dr Gordon Maden, a psychiatrist who over the course of 12 years sexually exploited his patients, mostly young men who were especially vulnerable as a result of having drug and alcohol problems and criminal records. The significant feature of the case from our point of view is that the patients had been complaining for many years. As *The Guardian* (4 February 1993) reported, other professionals had been aware for some time of the complaints but no effective action had been taken. One patient reported that he had been told to 'stop being silly' in response to his complaints (*The Guardian*, 4 February 1993). Even more telling was a comment reported from one of Dr Maden's colleagues to the effect that nothing was done because 'nothing really terrible had happened. . . . The addicts weren't too cut up about it. They had to deal with more degrading things in their lives. And addicts are cunning, devious people. To be honest, I felt they could quite easily manipulate him' (*The Guardian*, 4 February 1993, p. 6). Notice how, in this quote, they are not patients or clients but 'addicts'. They are also cunning and devious people. The originator of this quote unwittingly tells us why the complaints were not taken seriously for so long. If complaints are formulated as originating from cunning devious people who are not too badly traumatized, then these complaints are an exhibition of their pathology rather than having any basis in reality.

This is what we might call an *ad hominem* response to the complaints. They are seen as part of the complainer's problem and not a credible criticism of the care they have received. Examples like this imply that meaning in health care settings is not equitably negotiated between patients and practitioners. Patients may have an uphill struggle to have their voices heard. Even among well-informed, middle-class people, who would usually count as credible witnesses in legal and medical settings, and whose stories are likely to be believed, there are also many complaints. Again in the *British Medical Journal* (e.g. Greenhalgh, 1993, p. 464) there are tales of patients who had their questions dismissed brusquely at an outpatient clinic, or the woman whose concerns over a leg ulcer were met with the comment 'Look, dear, you go away and make up your mind what you want done and then we might be able to help you' before the irritated registrar disappeared out of the cubicle. It is not difficult, in talking to patients, to find cases like this, where they feel that medicine, and medical staff, have let them down through rudeness, unhelpfulness, or not giving them a chance to put their case. Equally, it is not difficult to imagine how this kind of approach can occur in the parallel world of nursing.

Whereas these cases are distressing for patients, they are often the easiest to put right, via sympathy, apologies or action by the professional bodies and the courts. What is somewhat more difficult to tackle are the more taken-for-granted inequalities built into systems of health and disease, suffering and healing, which, because they are so commonplace, are difficult to detect at all.

Let us explore further the possible taken-for-granteds in meaning as they show up in health contexts. The manifest position when nurses write records or discuss cases is that they are communicating about patients. However, it is important to reflect on all the other influences on language. As we began to argue in chapter 3, there is a great deal of institutional and professional practice encoded in language. When nurses talk at work they are not the sole authors of their words. As we also saw in chapter 3, there are preferred kinds of interaction and forms of talk. The unruly, joint transactions of therapeutic encounters are progressively 'cleaned up' by the actors, to yield professional narratives that tell us as much about medico-nursing storytelling as they do about the client. At the same time there is a whole store of linguistic devices that serve to produce the sense that our talk simply describes or reflects our patients. By contrast, we would argue, language is a fundamentally transformative activity.

The lens of language formulates people and their problems in various ways, depending upon the kinds of *frames* (Goffman, 1974) the actors are working with. For example, as we shall see later, studies of doctor–patient interaction suggest that there are complex rules governing the shift from an interpersonal frame of reference to a biomedical one. Language crucially informs the way that diagnoses are achieved and 'progress' is accomplished. This has important implications for ethnic sensitivity in nursing practice, as the dominant understandings of progress or desirable outcomes in Euro-American medicine and psychiatry will not necessarily be shared by other cultures. Understanding the language of health care is important in making sense of the critiques of medicine and psychiatry offered from anti-racist or feminist positions, where the frameworks and inferential structures of mainstream medical and psychiatric care are argued to embody white, male, middle-class assumptions and values (e.g. Parker *et al.*, 1995).

FORMULATING ACCOUNTS: THERAPEUTIC AUTHORITY AS A WAY OF EXPLAINING YOUR LIFE

One of the reasons why certain assumptions devalue certain groups of patients, like women, black people, 'drug addicts' and the like, or even patients who ask too many questions, is to do with the style of technical language adopted. In describing the clients or patients, the clinicians, observers, researchers and authors of records are able to deflect attention away from themselves. The operation of making things intelligible to the reader is often opaque. In a sense the writers of these stories about 'patients' are able to do what Haraway (1988) describes as 'the God trick', where the patient – 'the other' – is described as if from nowhere, as if the writer were transparent. As Fine (1994) puts it, 'Researchers/writers self-consciously carry no voice, body, race, class or gender and no interests in their texts. Narrators seek to shelter themselves in the text as if they were transparent (Spivak, 1988)' (p. 74).

Anthony Easthope (1986) argues that this 'clear and transparent style' was developed in the period surrounding the English Civil War by writers determined to argue clearly about religious and political issues. It purports to be 'styleless, a clear window on reality that presents the truth nakedly and objectively as it is without any subjective feeling or attitude getting in the way' (Easthope, 1986, p. 79). This mode of writing, in medico-nursing records and in social science is pre-eminently about someone else, someone 'other' than the author. Fine (1994) describes how the process of research itself has been active in constructing 'others', particularly when researchers have studied 'marginal' groups like 'the poor', 'mental patients', blacks, women, people who've been sexually abused, one- parent families and so forth. At the same time the middle classes, elites or the wealthy have been relatively less investigated. On the relatively rare occasions when they are investigated, they are good at presenting a relatively unproblematic life narrative which reveals few domestic, work or interpersonal difficulties. In this context it is instructive that Thomas (1993) identifies many problems attached to interviewing senior executives who, in any case, are apt to regurgitate the company's official publicity material. So the 'others' in social science are disproportionately members of less empowered groups such as the ill, the poor or the proverbial undergraduate student participating in research to gain course credit in North American universities.

In addition to the technical and organizational reasons why the 'others' of medicine – the patients – come to look the way they do, there are a variety of informal processes that yield this result too. The 'othering' of client groups in medicine occurs partly in terms of the way professionals develop informal and formal diagnostic criteria and category names for patients, as we saw earlier in Becker's (1993) account of the characterization of patients as 'crocks'. The process of creating others is by no means obvious, even to people who do it. The kind of definition of an individual as an 'other' which is achieved in medicine, nursing, medical research and mental health care is partly the result of the investigative procedures involved. In this vein, Angrosino (1994) describes how researchers, when describing 'mentally disabled' individuals, often restrict their observations to interviews conducted in clinical settings and thus tend not to understand the person 'as a contextualised participant in a world outside the clinical setting' (Angrosino, 1994, p. 14). The tools of the trade, then, leave their marks on the warp and weft of the meaning that is constructed.

The approach of many of the authors whose ideas we have drawn upon in this chapter has been to treat the products of official discourse as problems to be investigated. That is how Angrosino comes to be critical of conventional accounts of adults with learning difficulties, or how Woollett and Marshall (1997) (and their informants) notice how medical understanding leaves out a good deal of the experience of childbirth.

A key feature of these approaches is the assumption that knowledge about patients is not achieved by neutrally describing the 'patient' but that it is created by and interacts with other kinds of social business being conducted in the clinical or research context. Indeed, there is some suggestion that the very categories of 'patient' and 'clinician' are afforded and sustained by this social interaction.

The kinds of understanding and meaning engendered in clinical settings have much broader implications for how clients or patients understand their lives. Medical knowledge or information they pick up from their encounter with a nurse may be used in the future to make sense of their own or others' experiences. This is of particular relevance for postmodernism with its 'emphasis on the constructivist and fluid aspects of how selves are created and enriched' (Wigren, 1994, p. 186). It is also important in terms of how the social sciences have long been recognized to contain a 'double hermeneutic' (Giddens, 1976) in that humans interpret themselves as well as the 'natural world' around them. Human beings are incurable interpreters, explainers and sense makers. They explain and make sense of life with whatever materials are to hand, from medicine, nursing or health visiting, common sense, friends, relatives and the media.

Thus, it comes as no surprise that individuals can be seen enriching their identities and giving meaning to their experience by deploying psychiatric or medical knowledge. For example, Karp (1992) reports on a group of people who attended a self-help group for individuals with affective or mood disorders. The group participants were assembling accounts of their condition from medical and other frames of understanding. For example, Karp (1992) says that one participant, probably in his sixties, reported the following:

> At first I thought I needed more sleep than other people. Then I realised that I had mood swings. Then I learned that I had depressive periods. Then I learned that I had bipolar depression. Then I learned from the doctors that I inherited this from my grandmother. This was a learning process that took several years.
>
> *(Karp, 1992, p. 149)*

Members of the group 'wanted to accept medical definitions of the situation while avoiding personally troublesome labels' (Karp, 1992, p. 151). Thus the people who are seen by nurses, doctors and therapists will in all likelihood have some story worked out already about what their problem is. This story is not one which is independent of medicine. It is built up of fragments of what they have learned from previous health encounters, friends, relatives and self-help groups or even television, magazines and newspapers.

Likewise, other groups of clients in receipt of nursing, medical and social care are active fabricators of narratives about their positions. Angrosino (1992) identifies a set of strategies that 'mentally retarded' (*sic*) adults use to construct their autobiographies: 'People whose self-image is ambivalent . . . select autobiographical structures that enable them to symbolise the conflict between their backgrounds and their current situations' (Angrosino, 1992, p. 195).

In some cases the strategies of employing medical terminology and theories are well developed parts of ex-psychiatric patients' self-management strategies. Herman (1993) calls these medical disclaimers. For example one of Herman's informants reports, 'I'm careful to emphasise that the three times I was admitted was due to a biochemical imbalance – something that millions of people get. I couldn't do anything to help myself . . .' (Herman, 1993, p. 314).

In addition to these more formally managed identities that some researchers have documented, there are many more aspects of the way therapeutic talk and ways of conceiving of oneself have colonized twentieth-century understanding (Rose, 1990). Miller and Rose (1994, pp. 58–9) detect 'the formation of a complex and heterogeneous "therapeutic machine" which has attached itself to diverse problems concerning the government of life conduct . . . its potency has lain in its availability to spread a particular way of understanding, judging and intervening over a wide surface of practices and issues'. In this quote Miller and Rose are describing how, as they see it, a whole range of interpersonal, organizational and relationship activity has come increasingly to be seen in psychological terms in the twentieth century.

In this kind of literature, like Miller and Rose's work, or in Karp's, Angrosino's, or Herman's, the meanings generated about human activity are seen as being part of the regulation of human conduct which the caring professions achieve. Even when people resist definition or negotiate their way skilfully through the experience of stigma, they are responding to meanings and definitions that have come from elsewhere. At the same time, in the literature we have reviewed there are often optimistic or liberatory assumptions that if we simply listen to clients, or enable them to unfold their own narrative, then this has positive consequences.

CLIENTS' NARRATIVES OR SOCIAL CONTROL: A STUDY OF PSYCHOTHERAPY

In psychotherapy especially, this enthusiasm for the narratives of clients has been particularly prominent. Based on the kind of work we mentioned in chapter 1, in which human life is seen as an accomplishment of storytelling, narratives and voices have been grasped as important concepts in psychotherapy and counselling, but even in other branches of nursing, researchers are seeking the 'narratives' or 'voices' of care (e.g. Johnson, 1993).

Nevertheless, we will stick with psychotherapy or counselling for a while, because it is here that the implications of considering human lives as narratives have been most fully developed. Given that nursing often involves listening to patients, counselling and reassuring them, our brief tour through narrative psychotherapy might be applicable to the linguistically or textually mediated reality of nursing too. Given that Edelman (1974) showed how easily we can redefine everyday health care interaction as therapeutic in its own right, it is important to understand this debate as it relates to what goes on in any health care context where the client tells a story. What we shall do is outline some developments of the use of narratives in this context and then go on to show how the novelty and liberatory potential of this new approach are not always realized.

As we might expect, authors whose work is informed by the use of narrative metaphors often have well-developed accounts of what the clients' stories mean, how they get produced, the dynamics of the therapeutic relationship, power in therapy, and the interpretations they can draw. Let us briefly consider some recent writings on this theme. Social constructivist, narrative therapy may involve 'the assignment of positive meaning to what appear to be negative situations' (Holmes, 1995, p. 441). The therapy process might be more of an art than a science – whereas Makari and Shapiro (1994) admit that clear, logical guidelines on what it means to 'listen' in therapeutic encounters are missing, they still advocate attention to the 'patient's' unspoken, perhaps unconscious 'shadow narrative'. Thus, unspoken, pragmatic communication can be made 'semantic, public and *open to dispute*' (1994, p. 42, our emphasis).

The self-aware, storytelling subjectivity of clients is frequently emphasized: 'Thus as part of their personhood the clients were conscious, and within that consciousness they were reflexive' (Rennie, 1994, p. 237). Note that even within this narrative-orientated genre of therapy, authors seem reluctant to abandon what seems to be a very traditional view of clients as having inner characteristics and properties – such as the familiar layers of the conscious and unconscious.

In this body of literature, clients are even formulated as having powers over therapists: 'Patients present with a set of pragmatic needs and wants and they teach therapists how to help them' (Gross, 1995, p. 182). Analogies are drawn with everyday conversation, which has the effect of making the process seem more equitable. The empowerment of clients through therapy may involve therapy itself being 'demystified' (Hare-Mustin, 1981; De Varis, 1994, p. 592) so they can make informed choices. Moreover, 'The process of effective psychotherapy gives considerable power and respect to the patient' (De Varis, 1994, p. 592). Indeed, even the well-known critiques of psychotherapy as an abuse of power, by Jeffrey Masson (1989; 1994) can apparently be neutralized from within this perspective, according to some more optimistic advocates. For example, Owen (1995, p. 105) advocates 'self-realization' whereby the clients have a knowledge of the field and are competent to judge the quality of the therapeutic relationship in which they participate. The therapeutic mainstay of 'empathy' is being increasingly reconceptualized in linguistic terms which emphasize the 'co-creation of shared meanings' (Snyder, 1995, p. 241) between family members in therapy and between therapist and client. There are exhortations that therapists be 'patient' when clients are telling a story (Rennie, 1994, p. 241).

So, the manifest position of psychotherapy, especially from the point of view of authors interested in new narrative formulations of therapeutic processes, emphasizes a virtuous mutuality and empowerment of clients.

We now turn to some of the criticisms that can be made of this kind of approach to talk and meaning between clients and therapists. It is our contention that the clients in this context are not as fully empowered and autonomous as we might at first suppose. The first reason is that the stories clients tell are not naïve constructions. They are precisely informed, often by versions of personhood, mental 'health' and 'illness' which have clear links with the versions already in use by professionals. The 'self-realization' that Owen (1995) advocates as a way of promoting clients' autonomy is surely mediated by a range of professional and cultural processes that undermine the sense in which the consumers of mental health services can be empowered. Clients arrive in a health care setting already having absorbed a great deal of the therapeutic way of assigning meaning and narrating their problems. Professionals may easily adopt derogatory forms of understanding in dealing with clients or patients. Michelle Fine (1994) argues that we can perhaps reduce the 'othering' process by 'rupturing texts with uppity voices' and probing the consciousness of those in a position of dominance. Sadly, the resources of meaning with which we give form to and with which we communicate our distress are not very likely to make our voices 'uppity'.

Secondly, even though the meanings generated in the story told by the client are being attended to, the therapist is still encouraged to take a more evaluative stance. The therapist's superordinate expertise is never fully erased in this literature. For example Rennie (1994) suggests that the client may be using stories to mask or avoid contact with 'deeper' issues (1994, p. 241) – this judgement surely consolidates the therapist's role as a superordinate judge of the proceedings. Clients' narratives are explicitly described as needing management by the therapist to move on to these putative deeper issues (1994, p. 242). So they are not just left to their own devices.

The interest in clients' narratives which has emerged in the literature on therapy and which is finding its way into studies of nursing is often rather vague as to the precise structure of what goes on in therapeutic encounters. Often this literature has been written by therapists themselves, who are understandably keen to promote the idea that they have enhanced a client's autonomy or done something beneficial.

A related area where we can get some clues as to the microstructure of health care encounters is the study of doctor–patient interaction. This has not usually been done by doctors themselves but by linguists or social scientists, who often cast a more critical eye over what they see. Our discussion will draw mostly on studies of doctor–patient interaction because this is what researchers have predominantly studied. What goes on between nurses and patients has, as usual, slipped below the line of sight. However, this is a useful body of literature to review as it is of more general interest to anyone who has to interact with clients, obtain their stories of ill health and act on the results. This encompasses everyone from nurses to social workers, health visitors and occupational therapists.

Work of this kind is important because it highlights the way conversational practice reflects institutional roles. This is especially a source of insight because some scholars have noted how the 'frames' or boundaries of how clients' problems are formulated work – for example the links between biomedical frames and psychosocial frames.

Generally, authors have agreed that doctors' talk operates within a biomedical 'frame' in Goffman's (1974) sense of the term (Coupland, Robinson and Coupland, 1994). Furthermore, doctors' handling of questioning sequences where patients are asked about themselves and their symptoms forms a primary instrument of interactional control (ten Have, 1991). The possibility of uppity voices finding their way into the process or records seems even more remote when we consider the form of the medical interaction in more detail, where it has often been noted that doctors are apparently able to impose a set of priorities on their patients (Fisher, 1991; Mishler, 1984). Doctors' sequences of questions are often of a kind that allows only for short factual answers (Frankel, 1990a, 1990b) and that the interaction sequences initiated by doctors' questions often have a three-part structure. The doctor typically initiates the topic/question, hears the patient's answer and maintains control of the process by means of a 'third position' assessment (Frankel, 1990a, 1990b; Mishler, 1984; Todd, 1984). In addition, question asking by patients has been noted to be 'dispreferred' (Frankel, 1983, 1990b; Todd, 1984; West, 1984). Despite all these suggestions that the doctor–patient interaction works predominantly in the interests of, and at the behest of, doctors, there is some evidence that patients are well disposed towards the controlling behaviours of doctors (West and Frankel, 1991). These examples come predominantly from medicine addressed to physical rather than psychological distress, and involve physicians rather than the broad range of professionals in nursing, psychiatry, social work, health visiting or even hospital chaplaincy who deal with everyday health care problems.

However, there are implications here for understanding health care encounters as a whole. The microstructure of these encounters deserves much greater attention from researchers addressing the therapeutic process. The grander narratives that clients produce are surely emergent properties of an interactive process which is addressed at only a general level in the glowing manifestos for narrative psychotherapy we reviewed earlier.

The picture of medical consultations presented by this kind of scholarship on doctor–patient interaction is rapidly being complicated even further, however, by new studies that detect the coexistence of several 'frames' in medical encounters. For example, Coupland, Robinson and Coupland (1994) emphasize the use of what they call 'socio-relational frames' in interactions they studied between doctors and elderly patients, which prioritize social relationships and psychosocial issues. This, the authors argue, fits in with the emphasis in contemporary geriatric medicine on relationships and autonomous living arrangements. This diversity of frames that doctors can employ simultaneously might signal a desirable attentiveness and flexibility. On the other hand it might be that their ready deployment of frames and registers of enquiry enables the controlling behaviour identified in studies of medical interaction.

This is not to argue that medico-nursing encounters are always managed by staff in a way that brooks no dissent from the patient. Researchers such as Tony Hak (1994) are at pains to point out how clients are able to retain some control over the encounter. A US study of women's interactions with their physicians (Borges and Waitzkin, 1995) provides the spectacle of women working in the encounter to get their doctors to adopt a *more* medical approach to their problems and prescribe them tranquillizers, despite the doctor trying to get them to 'understand that it isn't going to cure any of your problems' (p. 39). In any case, the work cited above does not represent a monolithic bloc of homogeneous findings.

Our purpose in describing it is to highlight the way that this literature brings to the fore the possibility that professionals, not least nurses, interactionally manage encounters, and identifies how they do this. This contrasts with the equity, empowerment of clients and mutuality asserted in much of the literature on psychotherapy. We would suggest, crucially, that this difference in emphasis reflects the orientation of different researchers as well as any difference between psychotherapy and general practice. Certainly, writers on psychotherapy have noted how clients may refuse or respond sarcastically to therapists' interpretations (Madill and Doherty, 1995). Yet the very fact that therapists are the ones doing the interpreting, empowering and so forth suggests a level of interactional management that surely demands greater acknowledgement on the part of many authors who are concerned with narratives in psychotherapy.

AUTONOMOUS PATIENTS? NEGOTIATING AND LEGISLATING THE MEANING OF DISTRESS

Thus, the possibility that texts might be ruptured by the uppity voices preferred by Fine (1994) recedes even more, because it is increasingly difficult to tell where such voices might come from, as interactions may occur so as to rule out much of this unruliness. Moreover, the uppity voices may even puncture the text to demand more medication (Borges and Waitzkin, 1995). The implications of this body of work for therapists, nurses and other health professionals are important. The analysis of the microstructure of interactions between health care professionals and clients involves taking very seriously how the people involved manage the interaction. In the eyes of scholars who analyse conversation these are not simply tellings of clients' troubles which reflect a narrative inherent in the client, but are carefully organized joint productions. Thinking in this way about the social meaning of everyday life has a long and scholarly history. Berger and Luckmann (1967) are credited with being the first to popularize the notion that reality is socially constructed, but it was many years before Tilley (1995, p. 5) foregrounded 'nurses' roles in negotiating "lived ideologies" ' in the hospital.

Key reference

To illustrate the way that diagnostic and therapeutic realities may involve contributions from many participants, let us return to the work of Douglas Maynard (Gill and Maynard, 1995), who provides an example that we shall recount in some detail. In reading the following, it is important to be aware of the issues we have raised above, as to whose story or narrative is being foregrounded, who is managing the encounter and how the meaning of a particularly problematic situation is being negotiated and constructed.

The background to this case is that Mr and Mrs B are attending a clinic for children with developmental difficulties. Their son, Michael, has exhibited a variety of behavioural problems and they and the child's school are concerned to get a more thorough assessment made.

As in our examples above, they are not naïve. They are aware that, previously, other professionals have hazarded diagnoses too, one of autism and another of organic brain disease, and they have read some popular literature on autism. Why, they ask, is there this inconsistency between the diagnosis of autism which the present psychiatrist, Dr O, prefers and what they have been told in the past?

(Segment 3A (II:59:16) simplified and adapted)

Dr O: If there's a really big neurologic disease. Okay. And it looks as if the parents are going to absolutely freak if I say 'autistic'. Huh HUH! I'll go 'organic mental disorder'?

(Gill and Maynard, 1995, p. 24)

So the inconsistency is to do with the anticipated response of parents to the diagnosis. There is, Dr O seems to be saying, a consistency between organic disease and autism, and she is almost talking as if she is letting Mr and Mrs B in on a secret, as if doctors tailor diagnoses to parents, and Mr and Mrs B by implication are not like the average parent who would be naïve enough to take diagnosis seriously. Mr and Mrs B, however, are silent throughout this sequence and do not acknowledge the punchline.

The interaction goes on over some ground that covers the nature of Michael's difficulties. Dr O believes that the behaviour problems are 'all secondary to what's wrong with the brain', whereupon Mrs B draws on her resources of meaning to counter-argue that with autism 'brain waves are normal and there's nothing really wrong with the brain'. Dr O responds to this by listing Michael's difficulties, such as hypotonia, abnormal EEG, possible seizures, mental retardation, behavioural difficulties 'that we call autism', learning and processing problems and variability. This reprise of the problems does not yield an agreement from the parents, so Dr O continues:

(Segment 3B (II:1.00.48) – simplified and adapted)

Dr O: All of those things are symptoms of the fact there's something the matter with his brain.
Mrs B: You're putting organic and autism together, aren't you?
Dr O: M hm.
Mrs B: Well, see now, on the report Doctor Kay said he didn't feel he was autistic. He was an organic child. Yeah, that they were two separate things.

(Gill and Maynard, 1995, p. 24)

So the inconsistency is still at large. The 'report' produced by 'Doctor Kay' (line 6) is evidence for the contention that autism and organic brain disorders are separable, especially in the case of Michael. As an aside, we should note that in DSM IV (American Psychiatric Association, 1994) autism is a functional rather than organic disorder, so Dr O is working to reposition the boundaries even as she speaks.

After this, Dr O explores another avenue of alignment. Perhaps the precise label is not important in itself, she suggests, but it will enable the parents to understand their son and enable him to get additional services geared to his special needs. In the following extract there are also contributions from Ms L, a speech therapist, and Ms T, from special education.

Dr O: Yes, but what I would say is that you shouldn't get hung up in this label business.

Mrs B: Yeah.

Dr O: That's nuts.

Mrs B: No.

Dr O: It's obvious there's something the matter with Michael's brain?

Mrs B: Right. I just let the word throw me. I was just relieved to know that this is normal and then I quit worrying about it – if it was or wasn't, you know.

Dr O: Yeah. That's right. So you know there's something the matter with his brain. We try to tell you as specifically as we can where his levels or functions are.

(Mr B):   M hm.

Dr O: The literature that will help you get services and the literature that will help you understand how he looks. The autistic literature.

Ms L: Quite.

Dr O: Okay?

Ms L: That's right.

Mr B: Hm.

Dr O: So I wouldn't argue with Doctor Kay – I'm not gonna argue with anybody because he obviously . . .

Mrs B: Well I just didn't know what 'organic' . . .

Dr O: It's confusing.

Mrs B: You know.

Dr O: Yeah, he is.

Mr B: Mm.

Mrs B: What he was referring to, yeah.

Dr O: But if you use the 'autistic' label it'll get you services? Mmm. You know.

Ms T: Yeah, more appropriate to him and his needs.

(Ms L):   Mm.

Dr O: Yes.

(Adapted from Gill and Maynard, 1995, p. 25)

What we hope the reader can see from this is how the meaning of a set of events, like the problems that the boy Michael has been exhibiting, is established. It is not as if the meanings exist somewhere in the conceptual stratosphere and are grasped by people trying to make sense of things. Neither is it simply a matter of some people naïvely applying labels to another group of people who equally naïvely acquiesce to the labels they have been given. In these sequences we can see that the differences between different doctors' diagnoses are part of the participants' concerns. Not only that, but the participants here are capable of a kind of ironic distance from the literal meaning of the terms. That is, they are talking about the diagnosis of autism as if it were the right tool for the job. Theories of autism in the academic literature, which would presumably be part of these clinicians' education, do indeed describe it in terms of brain malfunction. However, as the interaction proceeds these are progressively sidelined in favour of the more persuasive case that institutional arrangements will be better made to fit their son if they use this 'label'. As Gill and Maynard say, 'Thus in an environment of uncertainty and possible conflict clinicians may persuasively portray the appropriate label as one that will solve practical problems, not one which is necessarily technically correct or that is a pristine, objective reflection of the child's abilities and their relation to diagnostic categories' (p. 26).

However, there are some questions that might well remain. Are the meaning and diagnosis of Michael's problems equitably 'negotiated' or are they 'legislated'? (Mehan, Hertweck and Meihls, 1986). Has the institutional version of the child been superimposed over other possible competing definitions? To what extent was Mrs B successful in questioning the slippage between 'organic' and 'autistic' disorders? The issue of 'negotiation' versus 'legislation' is relevant to nursing practice. We might begin to think about the extent to which nurses 'negotiate' or 'legislate' the meaning of their patients' physical, mental, emotional or spiritual distress. For example, what about feeding an unconscious patient? Legally the nurse has a duty to care but is not able to negotiate with the patient. Or again, what about patients who request euthanasia when the law forbids it? How can 'negotiation' take place here? Equally, what negotiation exists when nurses ask patients about their religion but often do not know what to do with this information, particularly when it comes to caring for them?

CONCLUSIONS

Out of our survey of meaning it should begin to become clear that meaning is indeed a difficult concept to pin down. This chapter has attempted to discern meaning in nursing by means of exploring several strands of scholarship, both in the abstract, such as semiotics and hermeneutics, and the particular, in terms of studies of meaning making and negotiation in understanding health and illness, understanding health care practice and making sense of therapeutic narratives.

We are still left with the question of what meaning is. After all the material we have reviewed perhaps one conclusion we can reach is that meaning is recursive; it is defined in relation to itself. It is interactional, in that it can be recognized by concerned, competent participants in a situation – they can tell when an event or word means something, but may be at a loss to define what meaning is. Meaning is informed by the ideas, values, materials and resources that cultures or situations make available to individuals but this should not distract us from the way that people use these creatively on the hoof, as it were, to ad lib their way through health care encounters.

Meaning is also content rich. Abstract accounts of meaning are very difficult to imagine. Within semiotics, hermeneutics, psychoanalysis, Marxism and feminism scholars have been concerned with how words and texts come to mean what they do, and have produced dense accounts of ideology and unconscious processes, masculine hegemony and feminine resistance. However, these have proved difficult to map directly onto everyday nursing and health care practice.

Various ways of making meaning have been developed by and for patients, professionals and relatives. What we have attempted to illustrate in this chapter is that a variety of other processes intervene to constitute the person's distress, mediate it in therapeutic encounters and give it form and meaning. These may be local, in terms of what a particular encounter means, or global, for example in terms of what it means to be a good, professional nurse.

Some thinkers, especially in psychotherapy and latterly in nursing, have been looking for clients' narratives, therapeutic plots or informal scripts which guide people's lives or therapeutic processes. However, in looking at language in health care we should be aware of how interaction does not automatically result in the rendering of clients' narratives. Clients may just as easily be managed according to the staff's agendas and forms of interaction in which they have very little voice or power to create meaning. As we can see from cases of malpractice, or even studies of interaction between therapists and clients, or everyday medico-nursing consultations, it may be that the client's organized structure of meaning has little chance of breaking through. Optimistic claims that we are dealing with clients' or patients' own narratives are sometimes difficult to reconcile with the suspicion that in some cases the diagnosis and treatment pathway may be legislated rather than negotiated.

The intimate relationship between medicine and popular culture means that clients already come into therapeutic encounters with theories about how their distress makes sense, even before they have stepped through the clinic door.

People in health care encounters deploy the meaning of things in a self-aware, almost ironic style, as in the example from Gill and Maynard of how the clinicians negotiate their way through the different meanings that may surround a child's developmental difficulties. Rather like the insights from the semiotic and hermeneutic traditions with which we began this chapter, these examples indicate how the layers and functions of meaning may be multidimensional or kaleidoscopic.

Perhaps, in order to grasp meaning in nursing and health care in general, we should not be afraid of fragmentation and ambiguity. As the hermeneutic tradition shows us, the very diversity of potential meanings might be an asset. Indeed, Shotter (1993b) is concerned that we do not get seduced by 'a nice, coherent well-organised narrative' (pp. 127–8). This, he argues, does not allow a full appreciation of the context in which people are embedded and the way it surrounds us with possibilities. A therapeutically re-visioned story which has been crafted for the patient by nurses is not necessarily more true, even if it results in greater happiness. In Shotter's view it has become more *intelligible*, however. The theoretical traditions of semiology and hermeneutics encourage us to see this organization as always incomplete, always provisional. Meanings exist by convention or because they are the most persuasive of several competing meanings. Thus, we must grasp the diversity and ambiguity if we are to do justice to the things that patients and nurses say, do, write and feel.

Perhaps the most useful way of extending the ideas presented here is to focus more fully on how this intelligibility gets established. We would advocate further research on a variety of fronts, ranging from the study of nursing systems of organizing and establishing knowledge and practice, to clients' descriptions and explanations of their problems, through to fine-grained conversation analysis of therapeutic and diagnostic encounters, and lexico-grammatical analyses of nursing language. Clients' own meanings and those of nurses themselves are occasioned among a much broader set of narratives which are equally important and worthy of investigation.

SUMMARY

Taken in the social sense, meaning concerns how we give order and coherence to our lives. We have seen how the culture in which health and illness is experienced gives us a whole range of resources on which to draw to make sense of our distress. Meanings may be negotiated at the level of individual conversations. We have seen by means of examples of diagnostic encounters that meaning is a joint production. In addition there is the business of attributing meaning to one's life as a whole. In this latter case it may be necessary to think of broader goals and images that give form to the often burdensome responsibilities of nurses and other health care professionals.

The meanings of our illnesses are often firmly embedded in our social lives. As well as the strictly medical dimensions of disease, our social abilities wax and wane with illness and it is changes in these which are often influential in propelling us to see a health professional. Meanings are very often controversial. In psychiatry, obstetrics and gynaecology the dominant medical meanings have been under challenge from users' groups, and patients have objected to their treatment in organized and influential ways.

Even when it appears that clients are negotiating the meaning of their problems autonomously, we must be alert to the possibility that nurses are part of the wider system of guiding them and providing the spaces into which their distress can unfold. It may be that in some cases the meaning of illness, deviance or distress is not negotiated but legislated. Nursing needs to examine more closely how legislative its role in health care has become and whether it can take steps – even radical ones – to strengthen negotiation between themselves and those for whom they care.

REFERENCES

Althusser, L. (with Balibar, E.) (1968) *Reading Capital* (trans. B. Brewster), New Left Books, London.

Althusser, L. (1969) *For Marx* (trans. B. Brewster), Penguin, Harmondsworth.

American Psychiatric Association (1994) *Diagnostic and Statistical Manual of Mental Disorders*, 4th edn, American Psychiatric Association, Washington.

Angrosino, M.V. (1992) Metaphors of stigma. *Journal of Contemporary Ethnography*, **21**, 171–99.

Angrosino, M.V. (1994) On the bus with Vonnie Lee: explorations in life history and metaphor. *Journal of Contemporary Ethnography*, **23**, 14–28.

Bandura, A. (1977) Self efficacy: toward a unifying theory of behaviour change. *Psychological Review*, **84**, 191–215.

Barrett, R.J. (1988) Clinical writing and the documentary construction of schizophrenia. *Culture, Medicine and Psychiatry*, **12**, 265–99.

Barrett, R.J. (1991) Psychiatric practice and the definition of schizophrenia. *Dulwich Centre Newsletter*, **4**, 5–11.

Barthes, R. (1967) *Elements of Semiology* (trans. A. Lavers and C. Smith), Cape, London.

Barthes, R. (1973) *Mythologies*, Fontana, London.

Becker, H.S. (1993) How I learned what a crock was. *Journal of Contemporary Ethnography*, **22**(1), 28–35.

Berger, P. and Luckmann, T. (1967) *The Social Construction of Reality*, Anchor, Garden City, NY.

Bootzin, R.R., Acocella, J.R. and Alloy, L.B. (1993) *Abnormal Psychology: Current Perspectives*, 6th edn, McGraw Hill, New York.

Borges, S. and Waitzkin, H. (1995) Women's narratives in primary care medical encounters. *Women and Health*, **23**(1), 29–56.

Cixous, H. (1981) The laugh of the Medusa, in *New French Feminisms* (eds E. Marks and I. de Courtivron), Schocken Books, New York.

Comer, R.J. (1995) *Abnormal Psychology*, 2nd edn, W.H. Freeman, New York.

Coulter, J. (1979) *The Social Construction of Mind*, Macmillan, London.

Coupland, J., Robinson, J.D. and Coupland, N. (1994) Frame negotiation in doctor–elderly patient interactions. *Discourse and Society*, **5**, 89–124.

Crawford, P., Nolan, P. and Brown, B. (1995) Linguistic entrapment: medico-nursing biographies as fictions. *Journal of Advanced Nursing*, **22**, 1141–8.

Dahlgren, P. (1988) What's the meaning of this? Viewers' plural sense making of TV news. *Media, Culture and Society*, **10**, 285–301.

Davison, G.C. and Neale, J.M. (1994) *Abnormal Psychology*, 6th edn, John Wiley, New York.

de Man, P. (1979) *Allegories of Reading: Figural language in Rousseau, Nietzsche, Rilke, and Proust*, Yale University Press, New Haven.

de Man, P. (1984) *Rhetoric of Romanticism*, Columbia University Press, New York.

de Man, P. (1986) *The Resistance to Theory*, University of Minnesota Press, Minneapolis.

Derrida, J. (1976) *Of Grammatology* (trans. C.G. Spivak), Johns Hopkins University Press, Baltimore.

Derrida, J. (1978) *Writing and Difference* (trans. A. Bass), University of Chicago Press, Chicago.

De Varis, J. (1994) The dynamics of power in psychotherapy. *Psychotherapy*, **31**(4), 588–93.

Duck, S. (1994) *Meaningful Relationships*, Sage, London.

Eames, M., Ben-Shlomo, Y. and Marmot, M.G. (1993) Social deprivation and premature mortality: regional comparison across England. *British Medical Journal*, **307**, 1097–101.

Easthope, A. (1986) *What a Man's Gotta Do: The Masculine Myth in Popular Culture*, Paladin, London.

Edelman, M. (1974) The political language of the helping professions. *Politics and Society*, **4**, 295–310.

Ellis, A. (1962) *Reason and Emotion in Psychotherapy*, Lyle Stuart, Secaucus, NJ.

Ellis, A. (1976) The rational emotive view. *Journal of Contemporary Psychotherapy*, 8(1), 20–8.

Ellis, A. (1991) The revised ABCs of rational emotive therapy. *Journal of Rational Emotive and Cognitive Behaviour Therapy*, **9**, 139–72.

Emerick, R.E. (1996) Mad liberation: the sociology of knowledge and the ultimate civil rights movement. *Journal of Mind and Behaviour*, 17(2), 135–60.

Fairclough, N. (1989) *Language and Power*, Longman, London.

Fine, M. (1994) Working the hyphens: reinventing self and other in qualitative research, in *Handbook of Qualitative Research* (eds N. Denzin and Y.S. Lincoln), Sage, Thousand Oaks, CA.

Fish, S. (1972) *Self-Consuming Artefacts: The Experience of Seventeenth Century Literature*, University of California Press, Berkeley.

Fish, S. (1980) *Is There a Text in This Class? The Authority of Interpretive Communities*, Harvard University Press, Cambridge, MA.

Fisher, S. (1991) A discourse of the social: medical talk/power talk/oppositional talk. *Discourse and Society*, **2**, 157–82.

Foucault, M. (1965) *Madness and Civilisation*, Random House, New York.

Frankel, R.M. (1983) The laying on of hands: aspects of the organisation of gaze, touch and talk in a medical encounter, in *The Social Organisation of Doctor–Patient Communication* (eds S. Fisher and A. Todd), Center for Applied Linguistics, Washington.

Frankel, R.M. (1990a) Talking in interviews: a dispreference for patient-initiated questions in doctor–patient encounters, in *Interactional Competence* (ed. G. Psathas), University Press of America, Lanham, MD, pp. 231–62.

Frankel, R.M. (1990b) From sentence to sequence: understanding the medical encounter through microinteractional analysis. *Discourse Processes*, **7**, 135–70.

Giddens, A. (1976) *New Rules of Sociological Method*, Hutchinson, London.

Goffman, E. (1974) *Frame Analysis*, Harper & Row, New York.

Goldberg, D. and Huxley, P. (1992) *Common Mental Disorders: A Biosocial Model*, Tavistock/Routledge, London.

Greenhalgh, T. (1993) We'll serve you with a smile. *British Medical Journal*, **306**, 464.

Gross, H.S. (1995) Supportive therapy and the model of natural conversation. *Journal of Psychotherapy Practice and Research*, 4(2), 182–3.

Hak, T. (1992) Psychiatric records as transformations of other texts, in *Text in Context: Contributions to Ethnomethodology* (eds G. Watson and R.M. Seiler), Sage, London and New Delhi.

Hall, S. (1990) Cultural identity and diaspora, in *Identity, Community, Culture, Difference* (ed. J. Rutherford), Lawrence & Wishart, London.

Haraway, D. (1988) Situated knowledge. *Feminist Studies*, **14**, 575–99

Hare-Mustin, R.T. (1981) A feminist approach to family therapy, in *Family Therapy* (eds G.D. Erickson and T.P. Hogan), Brooks & Cole, Monterey, CA.

Harre, R. (1979) *Social Being*, Basil Blackwell, Oxford.

Hartman, G. (1980) *Criticism in the Wilderness: The study of Literature Today*, Yale University Press, New Haven.

Hartman, G. (1981) *Saving the Text: Literature, Derrida, Philosophy*, John Hopkins University Press, Baltimore.

Harvey, J. (1995) Upskilling and the intensification of work: the extended role in intensive care nursing and midwifery. *Sociological Review*, 43(4), 765–81.

Herman, N.J. (1993) Return to sender: reintegrative stigma management strategies of ex-psychiatric patients. *Journal of Contemporary Ethnography*, **22**, 295–330.

Hollinger, R. (1994) *Postmodernism and the Social Sciences*, Sage, Thousand Oaks, CA.

Holmes, J. (1995) Supportive psychotherapy: the search for positive meanings. *British Journal of Psychiatry*, **167**, 439–45.

Hudson, L. (1984) Texts, signs, artefacts, in *Cognitive Processes in the Perception of Art* (eds W.R. Crozier and A.J. Chapman), North-Holland, Oxford.

Irigaray, L. (1985) *Speculum of the Other Woman* (trans. G.C. Gill), Cornell, New York.

Iser, W. (1974) *The Implied Reader: Patterns of Communication in Prose Fiction from Bunyan to Beckett*, Johns Hopkins University Press, Baltimore.

Iser, W. (1978) *The Act of Reading: A Theory of Aesthetic Response*, Johns Hopkins University Press, Baltimore.

Jauss, H.R. (1982) *Towards an Aesthetic of Reception* (trans. T. Bahi), Harvester, Brighton.

Johnson, R. (1993) Nurse practitioner patient discourse: uncovering the voice of nursing in primary care practice. *Scholarly Inquiry for Nursing Practice*, **7**(3), 143–57.

Karp, D.A. (1992) Illness ambiguity and the search for meaning. *Journal of Contemporary Ethnography*, **21**, 139–70.

Kiecolt-Glaser, J.K., Fisher, L., Ogrocki, P. *et al.* (1987) Marital quality, marital disruption and immune function. *Psychosomatic Medicine*, **46**, 7–14.

Kleinman, A. (1980) *Patients and Healers in the Context of Culture*, University of California Press, Berkeley.

Kristeva, J. (1984) *Revolution in Poetic Language*, (trans. M. Waller), Columbia University Press, New York.

Lacan, J. (1977a) *Ecrits: A Selection* (trans. A. Sheridan), Tavistock Publications, London.

Lacan, J. (1977b) *The Four Fundamental Concepts of Psychoanalysis*, Hogarth, London.

Levi-Strauss, C. (1963) *Structural Anthropology* (trans. C. Jacobson and B. Grundfest-Schoepf), Basic Books, New York.

Lindlof, T. (1988) Media audiences as interpretive communities, in *Communication Yearbook*, 11 (ed. J.R. Anderson), Sage, Beverly Hills, CA.

Madill, A. and Doherty, K. (1995) 'So you did what you wanted then': discourse analysis, personal agency and psychotherapy. Paper presented at the University of Loughborough Discourse and Rhetoric Group, Spring, Loughborough, UK.

Makari, G.J. and Shapiro, T. (1994) A linguistic model of psychotherapeutic listening. *Journal of Psychotherapy Practice and Research*, **3**(1), 37–43.

Masson, J. (1989) *Against Therapy*, Collins, London.

Masson, J., (1994) The question of power in psychotherapy. *Journal of the Society for Existential Analysis*, **5**, 24–35.

Maynard, D. (1991) The perspective display series and the delivery and receipt of diagnostic news, in *Talk and Social Structure* (eds D. Boden and D.H. Zimmerman), Polity Press, Cambridge.

Mead, G.H. (1967) *Mind, Self and Society from the Standpoint of a Social Behaviourist*, University of Chicago Press, Chicago.

Mehan, H., Hertweck, A. and Meihls, L.J. (1986) *Handicapping the Handicapped: Decision Making in Students' Educational Careers*, Stanford University Press, Stanford, CA.

Meichenbaum, D.H. (1975) A self-instructional approach to stress management: a proposal for stress inoculation training, in *Stress and Anxiety*, vol. 2 (eds I. Sarason and C.D. Speilberger), Wiley, New York.

Meichenbaum, D.H. (1977) *Cognitive Behavior Modification: An Integrative Approach*, Plenum, New York.

Meichenbaum, D.H. (1993) Stress inoculation training: a 20 year update, in *Principles and Practice of Stress Management*, 2nd edn (eds P. Lehrer and R.L. Woolfolk), Guilford, New York.

Miller, J.H. (1982) *Fiction and Repetition: Seven English Novels*, Blackwell, Oxford.

Miller, J.H. (1992) *Illustration*, Harvard University Press, Cambridge, MA.

Miller, P. and Rose, N. (eds) (1986) *The Power of Psychiatry*, Polity Press, Cambridge.

Miller, P. and Rose, N. (1994) On therapeutic authority: psychoanalytical expertise under advanced liberalism. *History of the Human Sciences*, 7(3), 29–64.

Mishler, E., (1984) *The Discourse of Medicine: The Dialectics of Medical Interviews*, Ablex, Norwood, NJ.

Moi, T. (ed.) (1986) *The Kristeva Reader*, Blackwell, Oxford.

Molleman, E. and Van Knippenberg, A. (1995) Work redesign and the balance of control within a nursing context. *Human Relations*, 48(7), 795–814.

Ng, S.H. and Bradac, J.J. (1993) *Power in Language: Verbal Communication and Social Influence*, Sage, London.

Owen, I.R. (1995) Power, boundaries, intersubjectivity. *British Journal of Medical Psychology*, 68(2), 97–107.

Parker, I. (1992) *Discourse Dynamics: Critical Analysis for Social and Individual Psychology*, Routledge, London.

Parker, I., Georgaca, E., Harper, D., McLaughlin, T. and Stowell-Smith, D. (1995) *Deconstructing Psychopathology*, Sage, London and Thousand Oaks, CA.

Peirce, C. (1935–66) *Collected Papers* (eds C. Hartshorne, P. Weiss and A.W. Burks), Harvard University Press, Cambridge, MA.

Pomerantz, A. (1984) Agreeing and disagreeing with assessments: some features of preferred/dispreferred turn shapes, in *Structures of Social Action: Studies in Conversation Analysis* (eds J.M. & J.C. Heritage), Cambridge University Press, Cambridge.

Probyn, E. (1993) *Sexing the Self: Gendered Positions in Cultural Studies*, Routledge, London.

Radley, A. (1988) *Prospects of Heart Surgery: Psychological Adjustment to Coronary Bypass Grafting*, Springer Verlag, New York.

Reading, R., Raybould, S. and Jarvis, S. (1993) Deprivation, low birth weight and children's height: a comparison between rural and urban areas. *British Medical Journal*, 307, 1458–62.

Rennie, D.L. (1994) Storytelling in psychotherapy: the client's subjective experience. *Psychotherapy*, 31(2), 234–43.

Ricouer, P. (1971) The model of the text: meaningful action considered as text. *Social Research*, 38(3), 185–217.

Rodin, J. and Salovey, P. (1989) Health psychology. *Annual Review of Psychology*, 40, 533–79.

Rose, H. (1988) Beyond masculinist realities: a feminist epistemology for the sciences, in *Feminist Approaches to Science* (ed. R. Bleier), Pergamon, Oxford.

Rose, N. (1990) *Governing the Soul: The Shaping of the Private Self*, Routledge, London.

Rotter, J.P., Seerman, M. and Liverant, S. (1962) Internal versus external locus of control of reinforcement: a major variable in behaviour therapy, in *Decisions, Values and Groups* (ed. N.F. Washburne), Pergamon Press, New York.

Sapir, E. (1921) *Language: An Introduction to the Study of Speech*, Harcourt Brace & World, New York.

Saussure, F. de (1974) *A Course in General Linguistics* (trans. W. Baskin), Fontana, London.

Schacter, S. and Singer, J.E. (1962) Cognitive, social and physiological determinants of emotional state. *Psychological Review*, 69, 379–99.

Shotter, J. (1983) Hermeneutic interpretive theory, in *The Encyclopaedic Dictionary of Psychology* (eds R. Harre and R. Lamb), Blackwell, Oxford.

Shotter, J. (1987) The social construction of an 'us': problems of accountability and narratology, in *Accounting for Relationships* (eds R. Burnett, P. McGhee and D.D. Clarke), Methuen, London.

Shotter, J. (1993) *Conversational Realities: Constructing Life through Language*, Sage, London.

Smith, G.D. and Eggar, M. (1993) Socioeconomic differentials in wealth and health. *British Medical Journal*, 307, 1085–6.

Smith, R. (1993) On not listening to patients. *British Medical Journal*, 306, 410–11.

Meaning

Smythe, C. (1992) *Lesbians Talk: Queer Notions*, Scarlet Press, London.

Snyder, M. (1995) 'Becoming': a method for expanding systemic thinking and deepening empathic accuracy. *Family Process*, **34**, 241–53.

Spence, D.P.S., Hotchkiss, J., Williams, C.S.D. and Davies, P.D.O. (1993) Tuberculosis and poverty. *British Medical Journal*, **307**, 759–60.

Spivak, G. (1988) Can the subaltern speak? in *Marxism and the Interpretation of Culture* (eds C. Nelson and L. Grossberg), University of Illinois Press, Urbana.

Taylor, S.E. (1989) *Positive Illusions: Creative Self Deception and the Healthy Mind*, Basic Books, New York.

ten Have, P. (1991) Talk and institution: a reconsideration of the 'asymmetry' of doctor–patient interaction, in *Talk and Social Structure: Studies in Ethnomethodology and Conversation Analysis* (eds D. Boden and D.H. Zimmerman), University of California Press, Berkeley, pp. 138–63.

Thomas, R.J. (1993) Interviewing important people in big companies. *Journal of Contemporary Ethnography*, **22**(1), 80–96.

Tilley, S. (1995) *Negotiating Realities: Making Sense of Interactions between Patients Diagnosed as Neurotic and Nurses*, Avebury, Aldershot.

Todd, A.D. (1984) The prescription of contraception: negotiating between doctors and patients. *Discourse Processes*, **7**, 171–200.

Townsend, P., Phillmore, P. and Beattie, A. (1988) *Health and Deprivation: Inequality and the North*, Croom Helm, London.

West, C. (1984) *Routine Complications: Trouble with Talk between Doctors and Patients*, Indiana University Press, Bloomington.

West, C. and Frankel, R.M. (1991) Miscommunication in medicine, in *Miscommunication and Problematic Talk* (eds N. Coupland, H. Giles and J. Wiemann), Sage, Newbury Park, CA.

Whorf, B.L. (1956) *Language, Thought and Reality*, MIT Press, Cambridge, MA.

Wigren, J. (1994) Narrative completion in the treatment of trauma. *Psychotherapy*, **31**(3), 415–23.

Willis, P. (1977) *Learning to Labour: How Working Class Kids Get Working Class Jobs*, Saxon House, London.

Woollett, A. and Marshall, H. (1997) Discourses of pregnancy and childbirth, in *Material Discourses of Health and Illness* (ed. L. Yardley), Routledge, London.

Young, H.S. (1988) Practising RET with lower class clients, in *Developments in rational-emotive therapy* (eds W. Dryden and P. Trower), Open University Press, Milton Keynes.

Zola, I.K. (1973) Pathways to the doctor – from person to patient. *Social Science and Medicine*, **7**, 677–89.

KEY REFERENCES

Castro, R. (1995) The subjective experience of health and illness in Ocuituco: a case study. *Social Science and Medicine*, **41**(7), 1005–21.

Gill, V.T. and Maynard, D.W. (1995) On 'labelling' in actual interaction: delivering and receiving diagnoses of developmental disabilities. *Social Problems*, **42**(1), 11–37.

Glik, D.C. (1990) The redefinition of the situation: the social construction of spiritual healing experiences. *Sociology of Health and Illness*, **12**(2), 151–68.

McAdams, D.P. (1993) *The Stories We Live By: Personal myths and the Making of the Self*, Guilford, New York.

Radley, A. (1997) What role does the body have in illness? in *Material Discourses of Health and Illness* (ed. L. Yardley), Routledge, London.

5 AUDIENCE: WHO ARE WE TELLING?

AIMS

On completion of this chapter nurses will have a greater understanding of the nature and significance of audience in communication, in terms of both the writer's or speaker's influence on audience and audience influence on the writer or speaker.

The chapter aims to increase awareness of the way that meaning can be negotiated or agreed upon between speakers/writers and listeners/readers and to begin to differentiate the various audiences that nurses engage with during the course of their work, and consider how nurses themselves are audiences for messages from managers, doctors and patients.

Nurses need to understand more fully the types and functions of language they and other professionals use, and recognize both the controlling power of language and the powerful control of health care readings. This should extend to an understanding of ethical responsibilities not just as producers of nursing language but also as active audience members for that language. Making the wrong assumptions about the audience can have disabling and disempowering consequences.

Finally, this chapter aims to attune nurses to their responsibilities in the dual role of being an audience to, as well as performers of, health care language. Further awareness of both aspects of language engagement may bring about less coercive and more participatory health care.

INTRODUCTION: KEEPING THE AUDIENCE IN MIND

This chapter addresses issues that nurses should be concerned about when dealing with the various audiences of their spoken and written words, and, indeed, their actions or performance. There are audiences that consist of just one person, a group, or many (Willard and Brown, 1990); that are face to face as in verbal communication or the theatre; that are invisible or distant but anticipated as readers of written texts, or viewers and listeners of 'electronically mediated messages' such as with television, radio or computer (Moores, 1993, p. 2).

It might seem strange to include a chapter about audiences in a book about nursing. It is possible to scan the indexes of nursing textbooks or the contents pages of nursing journals without ever seeing the word 'audience'. This strikes us as a serious omission. The lack of attention that the nursing literature gives to this question is a serious weakness, which we hope to remedy. In order to do this we shall borrow from disciplines where the issue of audiences have been widely researched and debated, such as communication studies and literature. In these disciplines the question of how audiences respond and make sense of what they see, hear or read has been especially important to scholars. This is particularly the case in television where broadcasters have needed to collect information on their viewing public (Ang, 1991; Meehan, 1990). Nurses, up to now, have had no such need. However, as we hope to make clear, in modern health care contexts the question of who might be watching, listening or overhearing is one that nurses ignore at their peril.

There are two major ways of seeing audiences. One is to see audiences as passive receivers and communication as an essentially mechanical process. The other is to stress the active role of audiences as interpreters, reconstructers and message builders in their own right. The next task, then, is to outline these positions and describe how they have applied to nursing.

PASSIVE AUDIENCES AND MECHANICAL MESSAGES

The first and most classic position on the subject of communication is that audiences are relatively passive. Marxist scholars have long believed that the mass media manipulate public opinion, that popular music and films keep people superficially happy and prevent them seeking political change (Adorno and Horkheimer, 1972). The working class did not agitate for a share of resources and power because the culture industry had made society 'one-dimensional' (Marcuse, 1964). Contemporary critics point to people slumped in front of soap operas or helplessly consuming broadcast agendas which they are powerless to resist.

This may seem remote from nursing, but in a sense nurses too have been assumed to be passive audiences who should absorb other ideologies and ideas. In the mid-nineteenth century, when Florence Nightingale was developing training for nurses she considered it vital that nurses have a sound moral character and this was impressed on trainees who followed her model of training. Equally she felt it desirable for some medical education to be included. This was not so that nurses could be independent decision-making professionals in their own right, but rather so they could be the servants and helpers of their medical masters, the doctors (Valentine, 1996).

The point is that nurses have often been seen as a very passive audience indeed, who can and should be manipulated morally and educationally, and were seen in this light even by Florence Nightingale, one of their strongest campaigners and advocates (Holliday and Parker, 1997).

As we discussed in chapter 4, the meanings that speakers or writers attempt to convey are never watertight. Meaning transmission is a tricky business, because the readers or audience of what we speak or write can only ever receive an approximation of the meanings we attempt to convey. This sense that all or part of the message might get lost along the way was especially worrying to people in the electronics industry. It is no coincidence that early theories of communication from a source of information to an audience were developed by scholars in this field. Shannon and Weaver's (1949) mathematical model of communication stressed that what the sender intended would be subject to noise and interference like a radio signal, and the receiver's attempts to reconstruct the meaning would often yield a different interpretation: 'the message received can only approximate the message sent' (Willard and Brown, 1990, p. 41). Shannon and Weaver's theories and models were lurid with the hope of a new age of technology. They were geared especially to machine communication and mathematical notions of how information reduced uncertainty; the very sort of concerns we would expect to find in the science of military battlefield radio and remote-control weapons systems.

As we might also expect from metaphors with cybernetic origins like these, even at the time, many authors argued that they are altogether too crude to capture what it is that humans do when they communicate (Schramm, 1954; Dance, 1967). However, the model does highlight that there is an inevitable loss or transformation of meaning as the message is conveyed. Moreover, even though Shannon and Weaver were more interested in radio waves than human speech we can see how this potential loss of information impacts on nursing. For example, we know from studies of nursing students that they appreciate extra efforts staff make to explain things: 'I found this one physio that I've spent a lot of time with. He's been great, telling me about all the different problems, what they've done, and explaining it fully' (Dunn and Hansford, 1997, p. 1302).

So, although transmission models of communication like Shannon and Weaver's are rather crude, they tell us a good deal about how language works in practice. However, what these 'passive audience' models do not illustrate is what the audience does to make sense of the messages.

ACTIVE AUDIENCES AND MULTIPLE MESSAGES

At the same time as this passive idea of audiences was being put forward, there were many people who began to feel that being a member of an audience was a much more active process. Active audiences have been a central part of modern communication theory (McQuail, 1992, McQuail and Windahl, 1993). Here, researchers have been concerned with the resources that audience members can use to decode the communications they come across. In the study of literature, to go back to an example we used in chapter 2, Janice Radway (1984) detects the way that the readers of romantic novels enjoy such material because it supplies romance over and above what their husbands are able to provide, allows them a little time to themselves and provides some reassurance for these women that their lives in the domestic sphere are all right. Moreover, romantic literature allows them a reassuring sense that they can understand human nature – despite the different historical periods and parts of the world they are set in, the novels always present humanity in terms of the same tragedies, passions, loves and ultimately the achievement of a relationship or, better yet, marriage. As we mentioned before, the readers that Radway studied regularly talked to one another about their books and thus formed an 'interpretive community' who actively shared and constructed the meanings in the literature they read.

In the same way, nurses could be considered as an interpretive community in that they are actively making sense of their situation and collectively acting upon it. For example, if they decide their situation is intolerable they may take collective action. As one nurse reminisced to Russell (1997) in an oral history project, 'We had two marches and we made sure there was minimum staffing . . . When we did the first march it was the day of the board of governors meeting and as we marched out of the front gate we looked back, and they were all looking out of the board room [window]. So that was really my first baptism of conflict. The second march we had to get a police escort . . . We were protesting but we weren't militant. The nurses did get a substantial pay rise in the end. It was very good' (Russell, 1997, p. 493). These memories from industrial action taken in 1974 show how nurses as a group, in this case from the Maudsley and Bethlem hospitals, were hard at work developing interpretations of the situation they were faced with.

Industrial action is an extreme case of the nursing audience answering back to the management. Clearly there are many less militant ways in which the nursing audience can be actively involved in making sense of their world. One further example comes from the sphere of nurse education. In contrast to the old style transmission models of education, some authors are suggesting increasingly that nursing students should be active participants in this process: 'Students should be encouraged to recognise the influence they exert over their own clinical learning environment and to proactively work to create the kind of learning environment which will best meet their learning needs' (Dunn and Hansford, 1997, p. 1304).

Being an audience or interpretive community is not just about being involved as an active audience member. It is also about going beyond the information given in the message one receives. Let us take another example from communication studies. Henry Jenkins (1988) described the cult that has grown up in the United States around the popular science fiction TV series *Star Trek*. Fans hold conventions where, as well as the usual film shows, speeches and memorabilia stalls, they would dress up as their favourite characters from the series. More interestingly, they might also dress as characters who *could* have been in the series but were not. Equally, they wrote stories and scripts for episodes that had never been broadcast. However, among the community of fans, many people had clear ideas about which stories were acceptable and fitted in with the spirit of the show and which did not. They were thus able to evaluate one another's efforts.

In the same way, having undergone training and having worked with colleagues, nurses can easily judge whether a new nursing action is likely to be a good idea or not. In a sense, something is going on here which is similar to what Jenkins noticed with *Star Trek* fans. In an example cited by Pridham and Schutz (1985) a new nursing problem emerged, in the form of a woman who appeared to be suffering from inflammatory bowel disease. She was also unhappy with medical procedures, having a dread of injections, as well as being unhappy in her marriage and confused by conflicting advice from her parents. In addition she felt sad and helpless about her failure to improve. Like *Star Trek* fans using building blocks from familiar episodes, the nursing staff were able to identify the problems and develop solutions, such as enhancing her ability to cope with fear, to develop a supportive relationship with her husband and to develop a sense of mastery and competence. Thus, the nursing staff were using the material they had learned as an 'audience' in the past to make up new nursing interventions which remained true to the overall spirit of the profession.

Nurses are an audience, but because they are also active speakers, writers and healers in their own right they also have audiences of their own. Nurses are in a peculiar position. The idea that they are like an audience for films, TV or newspapers does not quite hit the mark. In the next section we shall deal with some of the literary theory that has attempted to deal with the 'instability' of who makes up the audience and what they are doing. Again, we are looking outside nursing for theoretical inspiration because the discipline itself does not have a theory of its own.

VARIABLE AUDIENCES, UNSTABLE AUDIENCES

The variability of who makes up a nurse's audience at any time and how audiences respond to nursing communication, makes it difficult to be conclusive about relationships that exist between the speaking, writing or performing nurse and those who listen, read and watch. As Shaun Moores notes, 'The conditions and boundaries of audiencehood are inherently unstable' (1993, p. 2). Kirsch and Roen (1990) account for such instability in the following way: 'For classical rhetoricians . . . the audience was a known, stable entity that a speaker could analyse, observe, and accommodate. Audiences of written discourse, however, are much less stable and predictable . . . Writers often have to imagine or "create" audiences, audiences that can include a variety of readers with diverse opinions' (pp. 15–16). In this sense, there are both flesh and blood readers 'out there' and the implied reader or audience in the text made up of 'a set of suggested or evoked attitudes, interests, reactions, conditions of knowledge which may or may not fit with the qualities of actual readers or listeners' (Park, 1982, cited in Kirsch and Roen, 1990, p. 14). While some, like Russell Long (1990), consider that writers wield the power to mould the reader to the role or identity they want their audience to have, others such as Barbara Tomlinson (1990) emphasize the power of real readers to influence what writers produce. Tomlinson attacks Walter Ong's view that 'the writer's audience is always a fiction' (Tomlinson, 1990, p. 85). Often we have a well developed idea of where our language is going. Broadcasting organizations and publishers conduct market research, and most writers and speakers have a sense of who they are talking to.

Whenever we write or speak, we do so with an audience in mind, even an imagined audience. In being sensitive to their audience, nurses may present a different spoken or written text depending upon whether they anticipate that it will be heard or read by fellow professionals, relatives or the client. Again, as discussed earlier, 'canteen talk' is often markedly different from 'professional talk' and follows on from a perceived change of audience situation. Nurses may be particularly sensitive to potentially critical or judgemental audiences such as nursing or medical management, hospital management, the law, and indeed the patients or clients themselves. Thus nurses may be extra careful with any information they commit to written text.

Having noted this much about what literary theorists have to say, we can see the subtle development of multiple or different audiences in health care settings. For example, the kinds of audience health professionals have to address change over time. This becomes obvious if we consider the changes that have taken place in health care in the UK over the past few years. Recently the picture of health has been complicated by the growing dominance of market rhetoric in health care, such that nurses may feel compelled to validate care in the language of effectiveness and efficiency (e.g. Traynor, 1996). Yet at the same time, with increased bureaucracy and the perceived inferiority of nursing records compared with medical records, nurses may feel that their texts are hardly read at all. Nursing texts may have a short half-life, yet the various assessments, care plans, day-to-day progress reports, summary reports and so on remain potent communications, as we shall witness in chapter 6.

Key reference

Health care professionals, then, have a variety of audiences to address. Indeed, it is possible to detect potential hearers and audiences in what some people say about their work. This is particularly obvious when we consider the conflict of medicine and management. For example, one of Traynor's informants said, when talking about attempts to measure the nursing process:

> people might say that's an incredibly crude measure, it nevertheless is one measure we can use in terms of did it take two nurses an hour and a half to deal with someone rather than one nurse ten minutes and you know that gives you some basic indicators to help you delve into the issues.
>
> *(Traynor, 1996, p. 329)*

In this quote we can almost see the speaker forestalling the hearer's criticism – 'people might say'. Indeed, Traynor provides examples of people who have quite elaborate theories of how the audience behaves, which enable them to be convincing with what they say or do in a health care context. One nurse executive showed how she was some-what hesitant about using the language of quantification in nursing, but felt that it could have benefits in soliciting the support of doctors. As she said:

> One of the things that happens in health care is that if you do all the stuff that is quantifiable, like the numbers game and number crunching then you definitely can prove something in the view, I have to say it, of men in the medical profession who think they own science and research, not all of them but some of them.
>
> (Traynor, 1996, p. 330)

Here the speaker is explicitly orienting herself to the audience she is attempting to persuade, to give herself a little more grip on the situation. In addition we can see that in order to have this persuasive power it has to be a certain kind of information – one that fits in with the standards of objectivity and science.

Whatever is produced by way of language relating to people's lives, illnesses and ailments is structured in dominance. That is, there is an often unspoken assumption that the audience will prefer some kinds of information and not others. Holbrook (1995) describes how she began encouraging a client to keep a journal of her domestic duties and childcare activities ten years previously but did not believe that it would ever find an interested audience. It is only with the recent interest in people's personal documents as a topic for research that this particular narrative has found an appreciative audience. This hierarchy of information is not unique to nursing or even health care as a whole. We can see hierarchies like this working in mass commu-nications too, where scholars have long noted that people do not mind admitting to watching the news, but are sometimes apologetic about watching soap operas (Alasuutari, 1992). Nurses may be proud of what they have learned from the technical literature of the discipline, but less happy to admit listening to canteen gossip. And yet both the solitary seeker after knowledge and the gossip monger are engaged in a profoundly social process. As Asbach and Scherer (1994) put it,

> through human interaction the inner life becomes transformed into social experiences and systems and, conversely, group experience comes to be personally and internally represented. The two dimen-sions of inner and group life are linked by an interface, a network-system . . . consisting of verbal and non-verbal interactions linking members of a group. (p. 13)

In the next section, we shall look in more detail at attempts to make sense of the social nature of audiences.

TEXTUAL COMMUNITIES AND POWERFUL READINGS

As with the idea of a single author, discussed in chapter 2, the dominant view of a reading audience is that of a 'solitary reader' (Long, 1994, p. 182). But as Long is keen to argue, reading is as much a social and collective process as writing. She notes that, in art, people reading are depicted on their own, reading in isolation, and counters such notions by arguing that not only are people socialized into reading, but that 'the habit of reading is profoundly social' (Long, p. 193). In effect, reading is something that people do together: 'As midcentury American empirical studies of adult reading show, social isolation depresses readership, and social involvement encourages it. Most readers need the support of talk with other readers, the participation in a social milieu in which books are "in the air" ' (Long, p. 193).

In nursing, we can see 'textual communities' (Brian Stock, cited in Long, 1994, p. 195) operating in the way nurses discuss with each other previously written notes, assessments and reports. Case conferences may be seen as a collective reading of the patient or client. A variety of readings of all the various spoken and written information to date are offered. Of course, one may feel that the most powerful reading comes from the most powerful members, such as doctors. One wonders how far nurses become a non-reciprocal or passive audience to the empowered medical reading, and whether 'textual community' is misplaced in this context. Ian Angus (1994) writes that 'the ideal of reciprocity seems essential to rule by the people' (p. 233). He bemoans the fact that

> The tendency of the most significant contemporary communication systems is to produce audiences without this capacity. Audiences tend to remain simply audiences; that is, communication systems tend to sever audiences from reciprocal production of social knowledge and engagement in decision making. (p. 233)

Perhaps, for nurses, and indeed clients, case conferences can, at their worst, become like sitting in front of a television while the doctor gives his or her reading of the situation, while maintaining that bogus involvement of gaze and address: 'Hey, don't go away now! We *really* want to know what you think about this.'

At the same time, group activities like case conferences and management meetings may involve nurses being the audience for other participants who are keen to deflect blame away from themselves. The problems thus may be deflected towards the least powerful group present, which is often the nurses. Especially as they usually spend more time with patients. This process of defining the problem as lying with someone else has often been noted in studies of group behaviour at work (Hinshelwood, 1987; Morgan and Thomas, 1996). Being a member of an audience, then, is not always a pleasant experience.

To sum up, there are some powerful tendencies at work trying to make sure nurses as an audience cannot answer back. As education gets more technological, and health care more financially dominated, the opportunities to talk back are increasingly restricted. That is why it is vital to follow Elizabeth Long's lead and consider the audience not as a set of isolated readers or listeners but as a group of people who can rely on one another for support rather than passively receive the instructions of more powerful groups. Even more importantly, the bases for people's self definition change in groups. Personal identity gives way to social identity . . . in groups there are . . . new identity possibilities . . . [people] can switch on these identities in appropriate situations . . . adjust their sense of identity, their thoughts and their behaviours to match their collectively defined attributes of their social groups. People take on the group characteristics and make these their own, at any rate for the time being, to a greater or lesser extent.

(Tajfel and Turner 1979, pp. 33–5)

Now we have established that a crucial aspect of the audience is to do with social groups, it becomes easier to see what we mean when we say that the audience is *active* as a group of interpreters, sense makers and people who go beyond the information given. As we have seen also, there is not always a place for this activity to bear fruit. Nurses are sometimes constrained by conventions and occupational hierarchies. In the next section, then, we shall revisit the idea of an active audience and draw in some further insights from literary studies to establish more clearly how it is that nurses can be active participants.

THE ACTIVE AUDIENCE REVISISTED

In message reception readers or the audience are active participants. They are not passive: 'The constant process of making arguments is rhetorical. One side of rhetoric is persuading . . . Another side is being persuaded . . . an audience is active not simply the passive recipient' (Scott, cited in Enos, 1990, p. 99). What nurses say or write is one side of the equation. What the readers or audience of such communications think about what is said or written is the other side. In other words, there is an onus or responsibility to be placed not just on the speaker or writer but also on the listener or reader in terms of communicating care. So far we have argued as if nurses were a fairly consistent and agreeable group who tended to support one another's positions and interpretations, as the term 'interpretive community' implies. As anyone knows who has spent much time in a work setting, this is far from the case. Often members of professional groups will disagree, both privately and in public. Members of interpretive communities speak to and hear one another as well as interpreting messages that come from elsewhere.

This disagreement does not invalidate the ideas of textual and interpretive communities which we have outlined. In fact it is this disagreement which most clearly marks out the professional identity of nurses. For example, in the scenario involving 'Bill' in chapter 4, when a nurse says, 'Watch out for Bill – he can be very difficult', the nurse who receives this information should be highly sceptical of the foundations for this commentary. Rather than trying to locate exactly what is difficult about Bill and thinking, for example, 'He isn't speaking very much. Yes, Bill is very difficult – he doesn't speak', the nurse should call into question the statement that Bill is 'difficult'. She might ask the other nurse, 'Why do you think Bill is difficult?' This might draw more specific information and allow interrogation of the term 'difficult'. If she knows that the statement is unwarranted she might offer an alternative statement or rejoinder such as, 'I've spent a lot of time with Bill and fail to see why you find him difficult.' Another example might be a nurse's statement such as 'John is a hopeless case. He cannot do anything for himself.' If the other nurse finds this inaccurate, she or he should say so, or write a rejoinder to such a view.

In this way we can move towards a dialogue of care. When nurses passively accept easy or lazy statements about negative aspects of individuals from fellow nurses, and indeed other health care professionals, or keep quiet when they disagree about such representations, they promote bad practice. The negotiation of meanings in nursing is dependent not just on the producers of nursing texts but also on the readers or audience of those texts. Striving for a unitary text which confers fixed meanings about an unchanging natural world will inevitably end in frustration. We need to grasp the multivoiced or polyvocal nature of life in health care more fully. Health is a joint process, where errors made by junior doctors who have been on duty for 60 hours are corrected by nurses, or where patients object to or fail to comply with courses of treatment whereupon the professional tries something else. This rough and tumble is part and parcel of health, as it is in most other areas of life, so disagreement, discussion and questioning can be as valuable a part of the record of care as agreement or consistency. As Billig (1991, p. 17) argues,

> **Human thinking is not merely a matter of processing information or following cognitive rules. Thinking is to be observed in action in discussions, in the rhetorical cut and thrust of argumentation.**

Indeed, this argumentative nature of sense making is present even when we are thinking alone:

> **To deliberate upon an issue is to argue with oneself, even to persuade oneself. It is no linguistic accident that to propose a reasoned justification is rightly called 'offering an argument'.**
> (Billig, 1991, p. 17)

There are some important points of contact between the rejoinders, disagreements and arguments we have just mentioned and the ethics to which nurses, in theory at least, subscribe. In serious cases of verbal or written malpractice, where a patient or client is linguistically incarcerated or abused, nurses should formally report that communication event. Terms of address and descriptions that are considered by the nurse to be offensive and damaging should be rigorously challenged. In this sense, then, nurses' ethical responsibilities extend to other people's spoken and written texts. To choose not to hear or see detrimental nursing language is deeply unethical. Nurses need to be responsible readers as much as responsible writers, and it is entirely consistent with the ethics of the profession for them to grow more fully aware of the powerful effects of their written and spoken argument or viewpoint. At the same time, there is an ethical value in sharing a common responsibility to be sceptical about the speech and writing of various health care professionals.

Up to this point we have stayed with the notion of nurses as a kind of audience; an audience that may confer, disagree or otherwise jointly produce an interpretation of what it sees, hears or does. Here again, however, the analogy of audiences for film, television, literature or theatre breaks down. Nursing, because of its highly active nature is a kind of performance too. However meek nurses may be in front of consultant surgeons or senior administrators, they are also involved in putting on a 'show' themselves in the form of day-to-day care for patients, and it is this performing role we will turn to in the next section.

PERFORMING FOR DIFFERENT AUDIENCES

Audiences can be seen as 'a kind of magnetic field . . . As we come closer to an audience, its field of force tends to pull our words into shapes or configurations determined by its needs or point of view. As we move farther away from the audience, our words are freer to rearrange themselves, to bubble or change and develop, to follow their own whims, without any interference from the needs or orientation of the audience' (Elbow, 1981, cited in Kirsch 1990, p. 227). The style with which an audience is addressed often depends on the relative positions of the players in the scene. For example, Ruth Wodak (1996) describes a situation in an outpatient clinic where the doctors on duty are typically young, inexperienced and overworked whereas the nurses have worked in that specialism for years. Yet the nurses 'are required to package their greater expertise in a way that does not threaten the doctor's overall authority' (Wodak, 1996, p. 171). Successfully negotiating fields of influence of particular audiences is a skilled process. Nurses need to be aware of the various audiences they address and how responsibly they do this. They also need to be aware of the various audiences they are part of and their responsibility to clap or protest ethically. On the one hand, 'A highly developed sense of audience must be one of the marks of the competent mature writer, for it is concerned with nothing less than the implementation of his concern to maintain or establish an appropriate relationship with his reader in order to achieve his full intent' (Britton *et al.*, 1975, cited in Mangelsdorf, Roen and Taylor, 1990, p. 244).

A telling analysis of what it means to perform as a nurse was provided in the late 1950s by Isabel Menzies Lyth (republished in 1988) in a study of a large teaching hospital.

> **Patients and relatives have very complicated feelings towards the hospital which are expressed particularly and most directly to the nurses, and often puzzle and distress them. Patients and relatives**

> show appreciation, gratitude, affection, respect; a touching relief that the hospital copes; helpfulness and concern for the nurses in their difficult task. But patients often resent their dependence; accept grudgingly the discipline imposed by treatment and hospital routine; envy nurses their health and skills; are demanding, possessive and jealous. Patients, like nurses find strong libidinal and erotic feelings stimulated by nursing care, and sometimes behave in ways that increase the nurses' difficulties: for example by unnecessary physical exposure. Relatives may also be demanding and critical, the more so because they resent the feeling that hospitalisation implies inadequacies in themselves. They envy nurses their skill and jealously resent the nurse's intimate contact with their patient.
>
> *(Menzies Lyth, 1988, p. 48)*

This might seem a little overblown, especially the item about the erotic qualities of nursing care, but this quote summarizes a good many of the feelings that patients and their relatives might have towards the nurse's performance. Thus nurses need to remember that a variety of concerned audiences stand in judgement over what they do, say and write.

So far we have considered the nature of audience in relation to nursing in rather general terms and alluded to the fact that some of the performances nurses may be involved in relate to writing. In this next section we shall consider this in a little more detail. Even though the audience is sometimes remote from the act of writing, it is nevertheless built into the act, as we shall see.

Literary theorists and students of communication tend to assume that communicating is a kind of free-form creative process where the writer uses his or her imagination as well as a vocabulary of stylistic devices to enable the transmission of meaning.

Most nurses, like most other people in the caring professions, will never have that kind of artistic discretion when writing in a work context. There will be conventions to be obeyed about what things are called, what kind of information is expected and how it is to be expressed. In particular, much information that is collected in relation to medico- nursing notes or research data has to go on forms. Forms are especially interesting to us because they build in a potential audience for the communication in a most concrete way. Often people who are confronted with unfamiliar forms, for example relating to health matters or welfare benefits, will be confused or uncertain. Uncertainty, and even fear perhaps, is to be expected when so many forms that are filled in by the general public contain statutory warnings about the consequences of not giving the correct information. As we have seen in chapter 3, forms both constrain and enable the kind of communication that takes place. As Jylha (1994) indicates, pre-set answers with yes/no categories or scales may be difficult for a member of staff to fill in. For example, she reports the dialogue that arose from a question on a form being filled in by a researcher. The question was

'How do you feel about your present health: Do you feel healthy?' The precoded answers on the form were 'yes' or 'no'. Here's how one of the respondents, a 71-year-old woman, dealt with it:

> Interviewer: I would now like to ask you some questions about your health. How do you feel about your present health?
> Respondent: I feel perfectly alright.
> I: So you feel quite healthy?
> R: Quite healthy. Right now I have no aches at all.
> I: How would you evaluate your present health, is it very good, fairly good, average . . .
> R: I would definitely say it's very good considering the circumstances and my age.
> I: If I asked you to compare your health with that of other people you know of your age would you say your health is better, about the same or worse?
> R: Well, I've got practical experience of it. There's no one who'll join me any more on my skiing tours to Lapland. I go up there every year but this spring there was no one my age or even a bit younger than myself, who would have come along. So there's no doubt about it, I am reasonably healthy.
>
> *(Jylha, 1994, p. 986)*

Here interviewer and respondent engage in a dialogue which eventually finds itself compressed onto a form. This final response that reaches the audience of researchers and clinicians does not reflect the process of coming to a joint judgement of what the respondent's health is like, replete with examples and reminiscences about holidays. The form then does not correspond to everyday reasoning about health.

Over time, as people become more experienced form fillers, it seems they develop a technique of seeing through the form to what the people who might read it will want to know. Rather than slavishly fitting the writing to the box, one official in a Citizens' Advice Bureau presented to Sarangi and Slembrouck (1996) a very different attitude to forms:

> I take a cavalier attitude to forms – and I think that the purpose of the form is to actually collect information but if you can't put it down . . . in the box provided just scribble it in anyway . . . even our workers have to have us tell them to take that attitude – they feel so constrained by the form – they are attempting to answer something that doesn't really fit in the box – so I say well you know just write across the box what you want to tell them even if it's not answering the question because that way you can't be accused of not having supplied the information . . . that the purpose of the forms is to collect information not to make it difficult to present it.
>
> *(Sarangi and Slembrouck, 1996, pp. 135–6)*

So here the experienced form filler has a different sense of audience to the novice. This person has a sense of the audience at the other end who will want certain kinds of information about the individual to whom the form corresponds. It is as if, when people start to work for him, they see the audience as the form itself, whose grids, boundaries and boxes have to be treated with respect. Eventually they move to a richer picture of the kinds of organization in which that form will subsequently function, to bring the client health care, welfare benefits and so forth.

In any communication interaction, then, the audience forms an essential component of the activity. After all, if what is being communicated is not understood in the way it was intended, the purpose of the interaction has failed. So, for good communication, the audience needs to be taken into consideration. In nursing there are many audiences, all with different perspectives, and all eager to be involved and informed about what is happening to them, their relatives or to the population generally.

Telling stories about patients is an important part of the professional management of people and their problems. The story says as much about the teller as it does about the person being talked about. In talking about patients nurses will tailor what they say to meet the expectation of whatever audience they are addressing. After all, various individuals, such as family members, social workers, user group members or even the police, will all have their own narratives or stories about a patient. Nurses have to present their story within the context of various audiences that have their own explanations or understanding of the patient which may be in conflict with those of the nurse, who needs to be aware of how various audiences will each construct their account of events. This itself depends on who they are, the reasons they have for being involved and the different perspectives they bring to a particular event. The way nurses shape their communication with an audience may demand a clear division between the different roles they have. For example, if a nurse and a policeman in an Accident and Emergency Department are friends they will behave and speak very differently to each other in their professional capacities when dealing, say, with a person with multiple injuries following a road traffic accident than they would if they were enjoying a social evening in a pub or club. Nurses during the course of their professional careers quickly come to realize that what is being communicated and the context in which this is done have a considerable impact on how the transaction is conducted.

The forms of language used and the types of interaction engaged in are to some extent governed by institutional rules, roles and constraints imposed upon individuals, though there is ample scope to bring one's own individual style to how communication with others is managed. Telling stories about one's work is further influenced by legal, ethical and professional demands as well as the technical nature of the words used to denote certain characteristics of people. For example, it is perfectly legitimate to discuss patients in the ward office, but it is regarded as highly unprofessional to conduct such a conversation in the supermarket, even though the atmosphere of a supermarket might be more conducive to asking questions and clarifying issues. Even the language used is governed by the context in which one finds oneself. Nurses may talk about their work in a particular way on the wards, but in a totally different way when off-duty. Equally, when in the clinical context there is a tendency to use technical language, such that patients with a high temperature are referred to as being 'febrile', while those with normal temperature are said to be 'apyrexial'. Even patients who know the meaning of these words but who ordinarily would not utilize them may feel quite happy to use them in conversations with nurses.

NURSING LANGUAGE AS A KIND OF PERFORMANCE

Despite the many influences that shape the type of language exchanged between nurses, doctors and patients there is a great deal of scope for communicating ideas in different ways, for instance, informal talk in corridors, 'canteen culture', and informal 'leakages'. Nurses will be influenced by the 'magnetic fields' (Elbow, 1981) of various audiences and engage in a wide range of communication which is both formal and informal. Sometimes nurses may interweave formal and informal communication. For example, a nurse taking a health history or engaging in some aspect of health education may decide to share with the patient talk about holidays, family life or even the success of a local football team. These different types of interactional engagement are intimately bound up with the different uses to which language is put and the different ways it can be understood. The way most of us have been educated encourages us to think of some things as central to the illness experience – the precise location, intensity and timing of the pain, for example, is a worthwhile piece of diagnostic information. Other aspects, like holidays, football and who will feed the dog and take the children to school during the patients' hospital stay may need dealing with, but we tend to think of them as more peripheral. Consider for a moment what would happen if we did not have that intuitive grasp of where to put different kinds of information. If someone is suffering from appendicitis we would not usually write in their notes that they had a disappointing summer holiday – by everyday standards of reasoning it would not be relevant. However, it *might* have a bearing on someone who was depressed.

It is also important to note that in communication studies scholars are reluctant to talk about a single audience. They often prefer the plural term 'audiences' (e.g. Fiske, 1987). Translating this insight to health care, it reminds us that narratives about clients will make sense differently to different audiences or interest groups. For example, diagnostic categories in mental health may seem mundane to mental health staff, but can have very negative implications as far as patients are concerned (Herman, 1993; Herman and Musolf, 1998). Equally, some clients may be very keen to obtain a medically sanctioned name for their problems, as the debates over seasonal affective disorder and chronic fatigue syndrome have shown. So the use to which language is put is dependent on the expectations and needs of the hearer and the interpretation they put on what has been said.

As we have seen, the way stories are received and understood has been addressed in literary theory, linguistics, psychology and cultural studies, where there now exists a lively literature about how audiences make sense of texts. Audience interpretation can be diverse. For example, a single play like *The Merchant of Venice* has been interpreted in many ways over the centuries and doubtless will continue to be interpreted differently in the future. Different generations of actors have created very different interpretations of the characters, for example as tragic or evil, stately or down-at-heel. This process of the performer providing an *interpretation* of the underlying text occurs in other performing arts, such as when we speak of dancers interpreting music.

Using this as an analogy, let us apply it to the problem of how sense is made of language in nursing. In particular, we would like to stress the necessity of practising sceptical reading. Sceptical reading involves a suspicion of the inevitable reverbalizations that records have been through, and an awareness of the consequences in terms of how language may incarcerate or entrap patients. Nursing records are not somehow naturally authoritative, but this authority is accomplished through the contexts in which they are used.

It is by subjecting the language used in written nursing reports, which might appear to be ostensibly written about the patient, to intensive scrutiny that we begin to understand the many functions that a particular narrative can serve. A nursing narrative is written by a nurse about a particular event that she or he deems to be sufficiently important to record. Nurses select the event, imbue it with importance and relevance and write about it in such a way that other nurses will see and appreciate the reasons for selecting and writing on this event. The nurse will seek to justify why certain actions were taken, or that he or she was sufficiently astute to recognize signs of the patient either improving, deteriorating or remaining the same. In taking particular actions the nurse is confirming that she or he took the proper course of action appropriate to accepted good nursing practice. Even though this narrative is about the patient it also serves the purpose of reaffirming to colleagues that the writer is a conscientious and competent nurse. Thus, we could say that a great deal of nursing language is *reflexive*. That is, nursing language and actions address the nurse who performs them as well as an audience of patients and fellow health professionals.

This reflexive quality of language has been noted in differing settings by philosophers and sociologists. As Garfinkel (1984) noted, reasoning – and the language in which it is expressed – is shaped by the organization of activities it is involved in (Cuff, Sharrock and Francis, 1998). Let us take an example from Chapman's (1988) article about nurses in a therapeutic community. This extract occurred at the handover between two shifts:

Nurse: 'X the new adolescent certainly seems very strange. She fluctuated between being able to mix a bit and being socially isolated.'

(Chapman, 1988, p. 81)

This is a piece of reasoning which, as well as being embedded in the activity of nursing, is telling the hearer that the nurse has been watching for the right kinds of things and monitoring new arrivals in a responsible manner.

The example above was a verbal one, but written reports on patients could also be construed as a means by which professionals talk to each other about their jobs. In these reports nurses are making sense of the world in which they finds themselves, but much more they are inviting confirmation and legitimation of that world from their colleagues. That confirmation is provided when the next shift continues and builds on the narrative. Handovers between shifts are also examples of confirming behaviour when nurses describe their work to each other and one shift accepts the interpretation provided by the other. We can see this in the example below:

Nurse A: Bob's leg ulcer is improving. The dressing was changed this morning.

Nurse B: Good. How is the skin on his sacrum?

Nurse A: It's not broken. We're still turning him two hourly while he is in bed and standing him up for a few minutes at a time when he is sitting out in his chair.

Nurse B: Fine.

What is happening in these linguistic activities is that nurses are legitimating to themselves and others while at the same time making sense of their jobs. So the audience, those who hear or read what has been said or written, perform a most important function when it comes to communicating aspects of nursing work. It is through understanding what has been done, and accepting it, that the work is legitimated and validated and this serves an important function both for the narrator and the audience.

UNDERSTANDING AND SHARING KNOWLEDGE: THE IMPORTANCE OF CONTEXT

Understanding a narrative is a far more complex activity than might at first appear. Understanding assumes that what is being said makes sense and that it applies to a particular issue that one is concerned about. Furthermore, in order for anyone to be told something, that is, for them to be receptive as an audience, the language itself has to be understood and that requires having a great deal of shared background knowledge. To use a term from philosophy, this shared background and context is sometimes referred to under the heading of *indexicality*. That is, the meaning of many terms in ordinary language is tied to the occasions when they are used. Think of words like 'he',

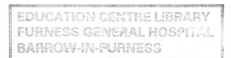

'she', 'it', 'that' and similar pronouns. When these are used, the speakers and hearers share an understanding of what is being spoken about. Yet, as Harold Garfinkel (1984) noted, any remark can be taken in a whole variety of ways depending on the circumstances under which it is used. The more knowledge, attitudes, values and beliefs we share with the teller the more accurately we should be able to understand what is being said. In order to get to know another person or establish a therapeutic relationship with a patient a considerable amount of information has to be obtained before we can make sense of the other person. The difficulty is that when a person is ill, injured or otherwise in distress it is difficult to establish a great deal of common ground with them.

In the building up of a body of knowledge about nursing, it is important that nurses share that knowledge with each other either in their basic education, post-registration education or day-to-day practice in the clinical areas. Many nurse educators have practised as nurses themselves, so the educational process for nurses involves nurses as both performers and audience. Like many professional bodies, nursing has a whole range of mechanisms for bringing stragglers back into line. There are a variety of post-registration or postgraduate courses which are increasingly and often aggressively marketed by a variety of educational institutions. If other members of the profession or managers encounter nurses who become 'out of date' or whose practice has been found to be 'dangerous' it is possible that they might be advised to undertake a course of study which will reintroduce them to the knowledge, values and attitudes that are essential in order to understand what comprises good practice. The process that is occurring in this context involves the nurse engaging in a discourse with fellow professionals in order to begin to acquire a knowledge and understanding that were previously lacking in her practice. There is a hidden curriculum to much retraining in that, in addition to the formal taught content, it helps orientate the trainee to what other members of that particular group are thinking, feeling, saying and doing. Whilst the academic or technical content may be quickly forgotten, retraining provides an opportunity to tune yourself in to the current mood and opinion of the group. Or rather, it enables 'out-of-date' nurses to know their nursing audience. Thus, there is a good deal more to being an audience than simply listening to the semantic content of the speech. It tells you that whatever you are listening to is a sensible thing to say in the current arena of nursing.

A consistent set of shared presuppositions and shared knowledge enables professionals to tell each other stories about medicine, healing and about patients themselves. As Hewison (1993) notes in her account of midwifery and labour, there is a great deal of emphasis on shared meanings among health professionals: 'Much of language use is built up on shared presuppositions and shared knowledge about social contexts; meanings by far outstrip the referents of the words themselves (Giles and Coupland, 1991)' (Hewison, 1993, pp. 225–6).

Thus, it appears from reading what we have put forward so far, that this community of speakers and hearers or audience members and performers in the health care community is relatively benign. Through education, argument and debate they can act so as to enhance patients' well-being. Within the context of nursing this may seem innocent enough but we only have to shift the context a little before a different picture emerges.

Continuing the example from childbirth which we began above, the usual language of midwifery, which would be unremarkable to someone working in the field, might appear more sinister to an outsider. As Hewison argues, much feminist scholarship on childbirth emphasizes something very different. On the one hand, the conventional medico-nursing vocabulary treats labour almost like work – with the uterus as a machine to produce the product, the mother as a labourer and the medical staff as supervisors (Martin, 1987). On the other hand, working from accounts by women who have experienced distress during and after childbirth, Kitzinger (1988) writes that 'Birth in western society has become an institutionalised act of violence against women, and postnatal depression is often grief that follows helplessness in the face of that violence' (cited in Hewison, 1993, p. 232). Here, the perspective of the audience hearing the 'language of labour' is crucial to understand the implications that they will draw from it. As health professionals talk mostly to one another, they are not readily exposed to more critical audiences who will expose the more sinister ideological freight that the language of health care conveys.

This tendency of professionals to be a very insulated audience – to listen to each other rather than to critical views from patients – was central to the problems facing psychiatric hospitals in the late twentieth century. Little attention was paid to how patients experienced being hospitalized or receiving treatment. Much that took place in psychiatric hospitals before 1960 was not communicated publicly. The inquiries of the 1960s and 1970s into what was actually taking place in these hospitals revealed that little communication existed between staff and virtually none between staff and patients (Ministry of Health, 1968; Martin, 1984). From these hospital reports it was obvious that different groups of staff did not communicate with each other, management was distant, and everyone assumed that all was well. In short no one knew what was going on, and they were unclear about what their role was. Among the many remedies that were advocated were more education for staff, more opportunities to discuss their work, more opportunities to share with colleagues what they should be doing and how well they should be doing it. In essence what this meant was to shift from a subservient culture to a linguistic one, where open discussions took place regularly and staff were held accountable for what they did. In short, staff had to become a more receptive audience – able to listen to each other and to new developments in their field.

Returning to the theme in the heading to this section – the importance of context – it is clear that context enables the audience to grasp what is going on. Equally, the context limits the way that people can make sense of the message. What makes sense in one ward may be incomprehensible in another. Again, we see this as an essential part of storytelling in health care and one that we cannot easily escape from. In addition, the stories we tell about healing, distress and disease differ profoundly from one health discipline to another, even when they are apparently concerned with the same problem. In some accounts the telling of stories is a profoundly fractured process.

In a sense, then, language and linguistic formulations perhaps serve as a kind of 'territory marking' and establish the contextual boundaries of different specialisms of care. This is especially so in mental health care. Samson (1995) presents accounts of various mental health workers about what they do and their orientation to their work. Unsurprisingly, his informants often told stories that emphasized their own domain of expertise. Psychiatrists were often keen to emphasize the insights possible from a biomedical perspective, for example: 'The only conclusion I've drawn is that the group of illnesses labelled schizophrenia is a biochemical abnormality. It's insidious, destructive. I think ex-patients have helped me to understand. I think with some of the schizophrenias, it has to be something wrong chemically. It has to be some sort of problem in the biochemistry' (Samson, 1995, p. 258).

On the other hand a voluntary-sector worker had a very different view of the issues: 'My philosophy is very much to work on practical problems first – to get people into accommodation, to get their rights and benefits, get them decently clothed and fed and then to look at other problems. Once you've done that a lot of people's mental health problems disappear' (Samson, 1995, p. 260).

Here, people see and communicate about things for which their domain of expertise equips them. Despite the contemporary interest in teamwork, when mental health workers describe what they do and the bearing this has on people's difficulties, their own approach often becomes paramount. This is what we mean when we talk of the 'territory marking' role of language. The action these linguistic formulations of their work performs for the workers is to stress how what they do is anchored, either in terms of biochemistry or in terms of some practical benefit to the client. In this way it is anchored also to the intellectual and professional context in which they work.

So far this might be innocent enough. Of course, what a physiotherapist says, for example, will make the most sense to other members of his or her specialism. People talk in terms of what they know, and this will make less sense to others who are outside their interpretive community or from radically different audiences. This becomes more of a problem, however, when the interpretive community becomes so encapsulated that it is immune from more critical voices.

An illustration of how insulated professional audiences can be from critical voices comes from the long-standing critiques of psychiatry. In

1961, for example, Thomas Szasz published *The Myth of Mental Illness* in which he argued that the concept of 'mental illness' is a metaphor and as such does not illuminate the experience or behaviour of the individual to whom it is applied. On the contrary it obscures essential features of the individual's behaviour and of the human situation in general. Szasz argued that the term was used to stigmatize deviants from social norms and to deprive them of their democratic rights and responsibilities. Farber (1993), on the other hand, believes that psychiatry's guilt was not informing people of their rights and not assisting them to manage their lives. The less people know about the workings of the social institutions of their society, the more they must trust those who wield power in it; and the more they trust those who wield such power, the more vulnerable they make themselves to becoming the victims of those institutions.

However, these critiques of psychiatry from otherwise respected scholars have had little direct impact on the day-to-day running of mental hospitals. It is interesting to note that the major contemporary impact of ideas from this critical tradition is not on psychiatrists themselves but on nurses (e.g. Hopton, 1997). Nurses – or at least those who write for academic journals – are a more permeable and receptive audience for critical ideas.

TELLING STORIES TO PATIENTS

We have established how telling stories to patients is an important part of nursing work. This has particularly been stressed in nursing initiatives in the community. In this context Martin O'Brien (1994) char-

Key reference

acterizes a great deal of the work nurses do as 'emotional labour' and sees the history of nursing as being characterized by an emphasis on these interpersonal dimensions of nursing work. In the nineteenth century, for example, nurses were expected to be 'cheerful, kindly, gentle, generous, courteous, discreet, grave, considerate, thoughtful, understanding, tactful, tender, calm, firm' (Garmilow, 1978, p. 115). The *Edinburgh Medical Journal* was reported by Abel-Smith (1975, p. 5) to have argued in the mid-nineteenth century that nurses should be 'endowed above all with that motherliness of nature which is the most precious attribute of a nurse'. This kind of orientation to nursing was observed in recent times by O'Brien, whose informants emphasized similar qualities in describing how they talked to patients. That is, the business of gearing themselves up to tell their stories effectively to the audience of their patients draws a good deal on their personal qualities and experience. For example, a district nurse said, 'we use past experience. We've brought up families and been a long time in the job. It just comes naturally, you don't think about it' (O'Brien, 1994, p. 401). A health visitor argued:

> When you're trying to get people to do something they don't want to do, it's no good coming on with the formal 'expert' style. You've got to play it like you do at home with your kids – get them to

> think they thought of it in the first place, then they'll do it even
> if they weren't interested to start off with.
>
> (O'Brien, 1994, p. 401)

This tendency to 'motherliness' in health professionals in their
dealings with clients can of course be a source of complaint too.
Care-givers interacting with elderly clients have been observed using
high-pitched baby talk, controlling institutional talk, short utterances, simple grammatical structures, interrogatives and imperatives
(Ashburn and Gordon, 1981; Caporael, 1981; de Wilde and de Bot,
1989). Moreover, there is some evidence to suggest that this use of
patronizing speech styles does not depend on the status of the patient
– the confused are no more likely to be patronized than those who
are alert and orientated. Rather, the speech style seemed to depend
on the attitudes of the care-giver – in a study by Caporael,
Lukaszewski and Culbertson (1983). The features of speech and
non-verbal behaviour – for example, high pitch, pats on the shoulder
and expressions like 'That's a good girl' – are not only perceived by
the elderly residents themselves as patronizing, but are also seen to
be unfavourable by observers (Ryan, Meredith and Shantz, 1994).
As Ryan, Meredith and Shantz argue, it is important that those
working with elderly people are aware of the tendency of carers to
talk in these ways and that some instruction on these matters is
incorporated into the curriculum of carers in training.

The problem here is yet again one that can be seen in terms of
audiences. This intuitive idea that health professionals have about their
audience – that they may be deaf, cognitively impaired or like children
– is at best patronizing and at worst can cause the very problems the
patients are assumed to have in the first place, as we shall see in chapter
6. Nurses here are 'talking to the wrong audience'.

The effects of this kind of patronizing talk are movingly described
by Albert Robillard (1996), who both is a sociologist and suffers
multiple disabilities. He describes people's responses to his anger at
this kind of mistreatment thus:

Key reference

> The response of my interlocutors to my visible anger ranges from
> 'I did not know you could hear', 'I didn't know you could think!',
> 'Most of my patients are stroke victims and have trouble under-
> standing me', to 'Oh, I am sorry, I won't do it again'. Most react
> to my outburst by ignoring me, leading me to see the ignoral as a
> further documentary reading of my symptomatology by my inter-
> locutor. It is a toss up if my harsh reaction will change the course
> of interaction. Frequently those who say 'I did not know you could
> . . .', or 'I am sorry, I will not do it again,' go back to exclusionary
> practices in a few moments.'
>
> (Robillard, 1996, p. 19)

It has been argued by some authors that institutional care encourages
dependency, by means of both overt and covert strategies on the part
of care staff (Avorn and Langer, 1982; Baltes, 1988; Wahl, 1991).

Being a 'good patient' – hence a good audience for the performances of nurses – involves being passive, compliant and docile. As Ryan, Meredith and Shantz (1994) say, 'the act of caring has been shown to foster dependence both by the message of incapability that it conveys as well as the very real reduction in ability that occurs when opportunities for utilising skills are decreased (Avorn and Langer, 1982; Kenny, 1990; Wahl, 1991)' (Ryan, Meredith and Shantz, 1994, p. 238). The language of the nursing home, then, in combination with the non-verbal and physical aspects of care is argued by these authors to be important in producing the disability itself. Moreover, despite the ethic of care in such institutions, the experience of being cared for is often profoundly dehumanizing: 'Older residents must adapt to a new set of routines, expectations and rules, frequently compromising or abandoning their own lifetime preferences, habits and needs. Further, they must make these adaptations from the socially inferior or less powerful role of resident or patient' (Ryan, Meredith and Shantz, 1994, p. 238).

In this section we have seen how a health professional's intuitive ideas about what makes sense to his or her audience are a double-edged sword. On the one hand there is a sense that they can make the communication more persuasive, but on the other there is a danger that this intuitive model of the audience seriously underestimates the abilities of the audience members.

TELLING THE STORY TO FELLOW PROFESSIONALS

The social arrangements between staff in the health service in the UK have undergone some profound changes in recent years. The languages of management and accounting have made massive incursions into medical and nursing practice. The types of information exchanged, then, have undergone a shift towards cataloguing the costs of care.

To illustrate this a little more, let us return to one of the studies with which we began this chapter, that of Michael Traynor (1996), who was interested in how clinical staff and managers discussed these very issues. Earlier we used his work to illustrate how people adapt their message so that it is persuasive to particular audiences. Now that we have discussed how audiences in health care context are multiple, how nurses may be both audience and performers, we shall emphasize how a grasp of these interactive roles is essential to making sense of health care.

In a sense the accountants and managers who play an increasingly prominent role in the health system have emerged as a new audience for nurses to engage with, as they insist that nursing must be provided in a cost-effective way. In his study of the relationship between managers and health care workers in some recently formed NHS Trusts, Traynor (1996) noted how keen the managers were for nurses to learn the new language of management. Thus, nurses claims about staffing inadequacies were seen as 'nagging'. Managers encouraged them, however, to learn to speak in terms of numerical information about 'patient dependency'. As one manager said in exasperation, 'I met the Day Ward Sister on my rounds and she was on about staffing and I said "you have evidence here of that" and she'd done no record of patient dependency' (Traynor, 1996, p. 327).

The managers saw themselves as driven into this kind of talk by means of financial pressure elsewhere in the system. As one nurse executive said,

> We get 12 million pounds from the DHA and they say to us, 'that's to provide your total community health service' – that's it. Bonk! I – let's be blunt about it . . . There's no point in – you would be foolish to ever think that money wasn't one of the bottom lines in most things.
>
> (Traynor, 1996, p. 334)

Thus, the manager's mission is to colonize other professionals who might not have the same world view. Their view is one where finance is central and anything else is 'foolish'. Interpretive practice then is a political enterprise, not just in party political terms, but in that one interpretive community often tries to prevail over the others. Ideas and philosophies based in the care and well-being of patients are going to have a difficult time competing for territory against a hard-nosed community of managers, accountants and politicians.

Whereas previously people involved in health management saw their role as facilitating the work of doctors and nurses, the orientation they adopt nowadays is increasingly one where they see their job as persuading the medical staff round to their way of thinking. For example, one manager told Traynor how he had embarked on a series of lectures to his clinical colleagues so as to

> tell people [staff] how we are doing, how we did last year, how many patients we saw, how that was better than the year before, what our financial position was at the end of the year, so that people actually know how the trust did, so it's first hand rather than a sort of a jaded documentary on Channel Four.
>
> (Traynor, 1996, p. 326)

Managers saw themselves as the guardians of true knowledge in the Health Trust, knowledge that was numerical and related to performance indicators. This was contrasted with gossip, rumour and 'invalid, subjective knowledge' which was 'politically motivated' and which had to be countered with 'the facts' – in other words, their view of the world.

In this example, then, language can be seen as enforcing a 'regime of truth' (Foucault, 1965) where views of the process of care are reformulated in costable, monetary terms. From this viewpoint a reduction in costs of as little as 50 pence a patient (Traynor, 1996, p. 327) may be touted as a major triumph. This development of discourses of the finance of care importantly talks this financial perspective into being. As Parker (1992, pp. 4–5) says,

> Discourses do not simply describe the social world, they categorise it, they bring phenomena into sight . . . once an object has been elaborated in a discourse, it is difficult not to refer to it as if it were real. Discourses provide frameworks for debating the value of one way of talking about reality over other ways.

To sum up what we have said so far, nurses and managers are an audience for one another, but what we have also been trying to show is how this relationship is not equal in that the managerial, economic talk is part of a project to colonize the health care professions and make them sing to the same tune. The discourses of finance established by the managers aim to colonize the minds and the working lives of clinical staff every bit as effectively as European settlers moving into Africa, India and the Americas. As Edward Said (1993) wrote of colonialism, the colonizer creates structures of feeling for the people who are colonized, so they cannot think of any alternative. Nurses, then, do not entirely make their own interpretive framework or interpretive community. It is made up of other people's meanings, commitments and structures too. This should underscore what we have already said about the importance of being a critical or sceptical audience. How far does the communicator want to make inroads into our thinking?

The study by Traynor (1996) illustrates a somewhat sinister theme in our discussion of audiences in health care. In the next section we look at the more benign attempts to make patients into a more participatory, active audience, and enhance the role of nurses themselves as critical listeners and active performers.

ENHANCING AUDIENCE ACTIVITY

Communication patterns between staff may be structured in very different ways. The apparently simple process of talking to fellow care workers or clinical staff about patients is infinitely variable. Despite this diversity, however, it appears that relationships can be detected between structures of staff roles and tasks and the kinds of communication that go on. In a paper on Swedish hospitals, Svensson (1996) documents how nurses talk differently depending on how tasks are assigned. In the more old-fashioned structure in the hospitals he studied, the doctors and nurses followed relatively traditional roles. The ward sisters followed the doctors on their rounds, informed them of the patients' conditions, noted their decisions about patients and then conveyed this to the staff nurses. The ward sister typically also liaised with the relatives of patients and handled external contacts. Under the new regimes that were being introduced at the time of Svensson's study, however, patients were looked after by means of a care team. This reorganization had profound effects on task organization and hence on the linguistic transactions between the staff nurses and others such as doctors and relatives. Nurses also were responsible for fewer patients and had a chance to get to know

Key reference

them more fully. This new regime of care, and consequently the new regime of language, was characterized by one worker in the following terms:

> We know the patients much better now than when I started, when one was called an assistant nurse. Then I ran about with drips and rushed to operations, hardly knowing whether Kalle Petterson [one of the patients] could stand on his legs, since that was taken care of by the enrolled nurses and nursing auxiliaries. Of course, I did my technical part, but the rest . . . And I wasn't along on the rounds . . . neither did the doctors ask for it then. Mostly it was a matter of medicines, papers and such things. But today the enrolled nurse also goes on the rounds. The whole care team tries to go along.
>
> (Svensson, 1996, p. 386)

Here patients are seen to be much more a part of the 'active audience' and 'interpretive community'. They are known as people and hence included. However, this new order had not entirely democratized the process of care, even though it had refigured the relationships between staff. When it came to medication, the nurses felt they couldn't blatantly recommend courses of treatment, as this could be seen as stepping on the doctors' toes. As one nurse put it, 'I think one says "You know he must be in a lot of pain." I don't say: "His pain is bad. He must be given a different pain killer." Perhaps I don't say it outright, though I may mean it. But of course I . . . actually could say it with the knowledge I have' (Svensson, 1996, p. 389).

Although this negotiation involved some of the staff in underplaying their opinions and knowledge, at the same time there was a developing feeling that the new system permitted a blurring of the boundaries between the nursing and the medical specialities. Moreover, under the new regime nurses sometimes saw themselves as the patient's defenders – trying to play a kind of advocacy role for the patients, and sometimes this draws them into discussions or arguments with the doctors about the course of treatment.

Most interestingly, the informants interviewed by Svensson who were nurses said they also performed a role as intermediaries between doctors and patients: 'For example, if the doctor does not appear on the ward in the afternoon to disclose the results of examinations, patients ask questions and wonder what has happened. In such cases the nurse feels it her duty to apologise for the doctor and give a plausible explanation as to why the patient has not heard the result' (Svensson, 1996, p. 391).

Nurses often occupy an exposed position between doctors and patients and their relatives and take on a shock absorber role. Obviously, this involves them in a set of linguistic interactions, but it also means that they are active in developing accounts of the patients for the doctors and accounts of the doctors for the patients. Thus, Svensson shows how nurses play a key role in ensuring that the construction yard of medical language runs smoothly.

The very fact that nurses have to take on such an exposed role in health care settings suggests that they are becoming a more receptive audience for patients. Indeed, it is possible to detect a movement in many realms of health care towards 'listening to patients'. Linda Gask (1997), for example, is keen to argue for the importance of psychiatrists studying personal accounts of sufferers, and Sarah Clement (1995) attempts to establish the importance of 'listening visits' in pregnancy as a way of making women less vulnerable to postnatal depression. This process of becoming more receptive to what patients have to say is not merely semantic. At its best it can incorporate some sort of emotional connection too. As Tannen (1989, p. 12) put it, this involves 'an internal, even emotional connection individuals feel, which binds them to other people as well as to places, things, activities, memories and words' – or as Lakoff (1990, p. 49) would have it, 'emotional connection, interest and concern' (Besnier, 1994).

The practical benefits of nurses being a more receptive, accepting audience are documented movingly by Weissman and Appleton (1995), who quote one of the hospitalized adolescents they spoke to as follows:

> The nurses here they understand my problems more and they help us. They don't get angry with you. If I get upset or something they won't get mad at me or anything. They'll just talk to me about what's wrong. And they'll understand and be nice about it. (p. 21)

FRAGMENTED AUDIENCES AND COERCIVE TREATMENTS

The example from Svensson's study we have considered above is about the professionals getting along together and effecting the complex social choreography of health care, as well as getting along with the patients. In this case the process has few problems. Despite the different views about the treatment of patients, they are at least working in the same direction. They are also employed by the same institution with a set of aims which are on the whole consistent, and, insofar as these aims promote health and minimize suffering, patients would probably agree with them. However, some kinds of health care may be conducted in situations that involve aims and policies that are much less compatible and which involve different agencies, legal and ethical frameworks, and conflict between staff and patients. This is most easily highlighted with an example from psychiatry. In the case of a study by Scheid-Cook (1993) the linguistic construction yard can almost be heard creaking and groaning as it struggles to keep the social processes of medicine on the rails. In Scheid-Cook's study, conducted in the USA, she was interested in the issue of outpatient commitment in psychiatry, where patients can be treated compulsorily without being admitted to hospital. This involves them having to attend day clinics and take medication at the discretion of the supervising clinicians.

Key reference

In this study clinicians were on the whole supportive of the idea of outpatient commitment (OPC); for example, in notes it was identified that 'Apparently, OPC is helping this patient in following through on his appointments since discharge from hospital' (Scheid-Cook, 1993, p. 184). This is a formulation of OPC which identified it as something that helps the patient. Thus, the author here has cut through the debates about the ethical desirability of compulsory treatment and neatly repackaged the legal decision as if it were a support to therapy. Indeed, some clinicians were dissatisfied with the legislation because it did not grant sufficient powers to the psychiatrist and the Community Mental Health Centres through which treatment was administered. As one said, 'OPC does not allow it to call the sheriff to bring the (client) to the CMHC and take their medication, the sheriff can only bring (the client) before the judge to be chewed out. If [the] (client) still won't come in, there's nothing we can do, there's no teeth in it' (Scheid-Cook, 1993, p. 185).

Here the reprimand from the judge (being 'chewed out') is regarded as a weakness of the legislation, that it has no 'teeth'. This lack of teeth was a source of frustration for clinicians. It was as if they wanted the law to allow them much greater powers over the people who were committed. The people who were being treated and their views were essentially marginal to the decision-making process. As another clinician said, 'Medication is what helps most of them deal with their mental illness and to stabilise; not therapy or talking over their problems' (Scheid-Cook, 1993, p. 186).

Earlier in this chapter we were concerned with interpretive communities jointly making sense of communications. In this case we have something very different. Here are some groups of people who are supposed to be involved in the same enterprise – psychiatry – but are saying and doing things that differ markedly from what patients might want. This is in strong contrast to the more inclusive model of nurses being a more receptive audience to patients which we identified in the previous section. This disjuncture is made even clearer when we consider the views of the patients themselves.

Many of the patients were critical of outpatient commitment. Whereas they cautiously welcomed it as an alternative to prison or an enforced hospital stay (p. 187), they were also able to identify a series of problems that it raised for them, such as the boredom and frustration of having to come to a mental health centre to more cogent critiques of OPC as a form of social control. As one woman said, when 'someone like her [one who is poor and a minority] goes against the grain, or has stress or money problems they get called looney and then are locked up' (p. 188). She said she had been given OPC because the judge was convinced that she did not need a hospital stay, but OPC created difficulties for her in that she 'had to make up an excuse for not coming to the mental health centre' when she had other things to do like family visits to make.

Some patients were aware that the authority of the doctors was enhanced by the use of OPC and that it forced compliance. Whereas the taking of medication itself could not be forced, OPC allows what Scheid-Cook calls a 'hidden interaction' between client and therapist where the client is relatively powerless' (Mulvey, Geller and Roth, 1987).

Now, what does all this have to say about the business of audiences in health care? One important lesson here is about messages that do not get through. The interpretive community of health and legal professionals can be seen on one side. They may disagree about how much power they need, but essentially they can work together and communicate intelligibly to one another. On the other side are the patients. They are often reluctant or critical and hence form an interpretive community of a different kind. In this example the competing points of view of staff and patients are especially visible. More importantly the accounts people give of their situation reflect their interests and points of view. The right to speak, moreover, reflects power and authority. In other words, 'telling' establishes and reinforces the hierarchies in which the participants are embedded (Bourdieu, 1992, p. 108). The authority of the telling comes not just from within speech, but from outside, from the legal system and from the training and experience of the professionals. These interpretive communities then are structured in dominance so that the legal-medical one is likely to prevail over the patient's perspective.

The social situation here also works to limit the audience for these different kinds of communication. Patients do not read their notes and usually do not overhear what professionals are saying about them. Likewise, professionals are not often confronted with the full extent of patients' complaints. This lack of communication is no accident. It is essential to the running of the system. We could say from a language point of view that the key feature here is that there are 'finite provinces of meaning' (Schutz, 1972) which clients and clinicians have. The structures of the law and the institutions create the spaces for these different provinces of meaning. These provinces of meaning often are sufficiently different that they do not overlap, but they are interlinked, like the pieces in a jigsaw puzzle, in order that the work of legally mandated mental health care can proceed. Indeed, maybe it is precisely because the views of the patients and professionals do not overlap that the work here is possible. Thus, it is not so much who you tell as who you don't tell which is significant in propelling the interaction. If the professionals found out what patients really say about them it would make their lives difficult. Equally, if patients discovered what was said about them they might be even more uncooperative and reluctant.

This example highlights the reverse side of interpretive communities and provinces of meaning. Sometimes it is necessary for them to be separate in order for the more coercive kinds of 'health care' work to carry on. This example also highlights why the issue of compulsory treatment is controversial. It goes against the idea that health care should be a consensual, collaborative process where sufferers and healers share the experiences and meanings as well as therapeutic techniques. It involves professionals shutting themselves off and insulating themselves as a potential audience to patients and their complaints.

As we hope to have made apparent in the last two sections, the more facilitative and client-centred forms of care involve a multiple, mutual acceptance of the audience role, such that professionals and patients can take it in turns to be performers and audiences. This is a model of care which is currently becoming fashionable where theorists of the nursing process have tried to emphasize dialogue rather than monologue (e.g. Geist and Dreyer, 1993). Understanding what the concept of audience means, then, can be useful in illuminating what goes on in both cooperative and coercive modes of care.

CONCLUSIONS

When nurses come to reflect upon their practice, a major component of their work should be how they have related to the various kinds of audience around them. Are they convinced that what they communicate is received as it was meant, is appropriate and ethical? Do they have evidence for a defensible approximation between the meaning sent and the meaning received? As we have pointed out in the course of this chapter, there are problems in telling stories about patients and telling stories to them. This is because, despite appearances to the contrary, there are so many factors that influence what is said, how it is received and what is meant. In nursing, one is always seeking to validate what is said. Nurses ensure that their message is understood both in what was intended and with respect to what the consequences might be. Patients, on the other hand, should be assisted to be understood. Restating, rephrasing and reviewing the statements that patients make helps to clarify what they mean by them. This can be an intellectually demanding task, but central to the practice of good nursing. In order to stand as true advocates of those in their care, nurses need to grasp fully their responsibilities as textual producers and receivers. If they do not take a principled and vigilant stand within the 'textual community' of health care, then nursing will continue to have a weak role in textual power play.

Let us now try to offer some recommendations for change and improvement in nursing. Firstly, being conscious of language is a skill which takes time to build up so it is important that health care workers regularly subject aspects of their work to scrutiny. It would be better still if we could enable this to be built into professional education and development, so that nurses have opportunities to examine their work in this way in the presence of a mentor or a Clinical Supervisor, who themselves have become more linguistically aware. It is possible that as part of their education nurses could examine their own nursing notes or tape-recorded samples of their conversations with patients and read and listen critically to what was written or said. From our experience in nursing education it is clear that nurses can be very critical of themselves, in terms of spelling or grammatical errors, how they sound, their accent, their incomplete sentences, the way they miss points that patients are attempting to make. The point of doing this is not to make nurses approach language negatively but on the contrary to improve their communication power for the future.

Secondly, we shall make a plea for universities and colleges where nursing is taught, and hospitals and community health services where it is practised, to create safe environments where nurses and other health professionals can regularly come together to discuss their work and any difficulties they may be having. All too often education and training are ghettoized into courses that last a few days and do not impinge on the rest of our working lives. One of the major sources of education, however, is ourselves. As language is something that fundamentally exists within communities, the greater the sense of community the more language there will be to study, reflect upon and ultimately enjoy. Rather than being peripheral to the business of health care, informal discussion is one of the major sites where it can be reflected upon and perhaps transformed. It is here that the critical voices we mentioned earlier can be sought out, attended to and mobilized by nurses themselves. Perhaps as an adjunct to this a certain amount of networking might not go amiss. The formal business of an organization is performed by means of informal talk. Colleagues help us much more readily with our formal work if they consider us to be friends who are concerned about their families and the fortunes of their football teams. Needless to say, the same is true of patients.

Thirdly, we would make a plea for nurses themselves to become more sensitive to language. In an ideal world all nurses should develop the habit of reading and paying particular attention to how different authors convey meaning, or how meaning is transmitted in the wider media. It is also important for nurses to contemplate who makes up their audience. Who do they speak to or write for? Imagine yourself on stage in an empty theatre. Now try to fill the seats with the audience of your various communications in nursing. Try to establish how sensitive you are to the various members of that audience.

Finally, let us note once again how odd it is that the question of audience has been left out of nursing for so long; for nurses as a group of people are constantly reading, listening, discussing and are themselves continually performing for audiences of patients, their relatives or even fellow health professionals. This continual process of reconstruction is an important part of what a nurse's identity is made up of. As Stuart Hall puts it,

Cultural identity . . . is a matter of 'becoming' as well as of 'being'. It belongs to the future as much as to the past. It is not something which already exists, transcending place, time history and culture. Cultural identities come from somewhere, have histories. But like everything which is historical, they undergo constant transformation. Far from being eternally fixed in some essentialised past, they are subject to the continuous play of history, culture and power.

(Hall, 1990, p. 225)

Thus nurses are continually recreating their identity and that of their profession through their listening, understanding, speaking and performing. This dynamic process of identity creation depends on nurses being both audiences and performers. After all, the profession is no longer as Florence Nightingale crafted it in the nineteenth century and the continuous process of communication surrounding and embedded in health care activities is the mechanism of change.

To conclude, we would make a case for nurses to attempt to be even more active as an audience and listen and read critically what fellow nurses and other health care professionals say and write. It is part of the ethical responsibility of nursing to try to intervene in other people's textual practice. It is important that the nursing profession thinks through the consequences of audience passivity. Being a passive audience means, as we have said, that a good deal of distress will go unchallenged.

SUMMARY

The issue of audiences is a diverse one within the language of health care. Writers often have an imaginary audience in mind when they speak or write and this influences the style and substance of their communications. Audience members themselves are active in decoding and interpreting communications so no direct links between the message and its effects can be assumed. Our ideas about who is listening or will read any communication have a bearing on how we will speak or write.

The cues as to how a message will be read may be ambiguous. For example, when confronted with an unfamiliar form, we may be unsure of how to complete the boxes adequately, whereas the experienced form filler has a well-developed idea of what the audience at the other end wants to know and will often appear to take a cavalier attitude to the lines and boxes themselves.

Language may be dressed up differently depending on the occasion. A nurse persuading a doctor may do so indirectly; a nurse persuading a manager may have to adopt a style of language more befitting an accountant than a health care professional.

It may even be that, in some circumstances, people's lack of communication is what keeps the organization going. In cases where patient treatment or attendance is compulsory, the fact that the staff do not hear the complaints of the patients may enable them to carry on doing their jobs. It is important in considering the question of audiences to be aware of what is not seen or heard as well as what is made obvious.

REFERENCES

Abel-Smith, B. (1975) *A History of the Nursing Profession*, 5th edn, Heinemann, London.
Adorno, T.W. and Horkheimer, M. (1972) The culture industry: enlightenment as mass deception, in *The Dialectics of Enlightenment*, Herder & Herder, New York.

Alasuutari, P. (1992) I'm ashamed to admit it but I have watched Dallas: the moral hierarchy of TV programmes. *Media, Culture and Society*, **14**, 561–82.

Ang, I. (1991) *Desperately Seeking the Audience*, Routledge, London.

Angus, I. (1994) Democracy and the constitution of audiences: a comparative media perspective, in *Viewing, Reading, Listening: Audiences and Cultural Reception* (eds J. Cruz and J. Lewis), Westview Press, Boulder, pp. 223–52.

Asbach, C. and Scherer, V. (1994) *Object Relations, the Self and the Group*, 2nd edn, Routledge, London.

Ashburn, G. and Gordon, A. (1981) Features of a simplified register in speech to elderly conversationalists. *International Journal of Psycholinguistics*, **8**, 7–31.

Avorn, J. and Langer, E. (1982) Induced disability in nursing home patients: a controlled trial. *Journal of the American Geriatrics Society*, **29**, 397–400.

Baltes, M.M. (1988) The etiology and maintenance of dependency in the elderly: three phases of operant research. *Behaviour Therapy*, **19**, 301–19.

Besnier, N. (1994) Involvement in linguistic practice: an ethnographic appraisal. *Journal of Pragmatics*, **22**, 279–99.

Billig, M. (1991) *Ideology and Opinions: Studies in Rhetorical Psychology*, Sage, London.

Bourdieu, P. (1992) *Language and Symbolic Power*, Polity Press, Cambridge.

Britton, J., Burgess, T., Martin, N., McLeod, A. and Rosen, H. (1975) *The Development of Writing Abilities (11–18)*, Macmillan, London.

Caporael, L. (1981) The paralanguage of care giving: baby talk and the institutionalised elderly. *Journal of Personality and Social Psychology*, **40**(5), 876–84.

Caporael, L., Lukaszewski, M. and Culbertson, G. (1983) Secondary baby talk: judgements by institutionalised elderly and their caregivers. *Journal of Personality and Social Psychology*, **44**(4), 746–54.

Chapman, G.E. (1988) Text, talk and discourse in a therapeutic community. *International Journal of Therapeutic Communities*, **9**(2), 75–87.

Clement, S. (1995) Listening visits in pregnancy: a strategy for preventing postnatal depression. *Midwifery*, **11**, 75–80.

Cuff, E.C., Sharrock, W.W. and Francis, D.W. (1998) *Perspectives in Sociology*, 4th edn, Routledge, London.

Dance, F.E.X. (1967) A helical model of communication, in *Human Communication Theory* (ed. F.E.X. Dance), Holt, Rinehart & Winston, New York.

de Wilde, I. and de Bot, K. (1989) Taal van verzorgenden tegen ouderen in een psychogeriatrisch verpleeghuis (A simplified speech register in caregivers' speech to elderly demented patients). *Tijdschrift voor Gerontologie en Geriatrie*, **20**, 97–100.

Dunn, S.V. and Hansford, B. (1997) Undergraduate nursing students' perceptions of their clinical learning environment. *Journal of Advanced Nursing*, **25**, 1299–306.

Elbow, P. (1981) *Writing with Power: Techniques for Mastering the Writing Process*, Oxford University Press, New York.

Enos, T. (1990) 'An eternal golden braid': rhetor as audience, audience as rhetor, in *A Sense of Audience in Written Communication. Written Communication Annual: An International Survey of Research and Theory*, vol. 5 (eds G. Kirsch and D.H. Roen), Sage, London, pp. 99–114.

Farber, S. (1993) *Madness, Heresy and the Rumour of Angels*, Open Court, Chicago and La Salle, IL.

Fiske, J. (1987) *Television Culture*, Methuen, London.

Foucault, M. (1965) *Madness and Civilisation: A History of Insanity in the Age of Reason*, Pantheon, New York.

Garfinkel, H. (1984) *Studies in Ethnomethodology*, Polity Press, Cambridge.

Garmilow, E. (1978) Sexual division of labour: the case of nursing, in *Feminism and Materialism: Women and Modes of Production* (eds A. Kuhn and A.M. Wolpe), Routledge, London.

Gask, L. (1997) Listening to patients. *British Journal of Psychiatry*, **171**, 301–2.

Geist, P. and Dreyer, J. (1993) The demise of dialogue: a critique of medical encounter ideology. *Western Journal of Communication*, 57, 233–46.

Giles, H. and Coupland, N. (1991) *Language: Contexts and Consequences*, Open University Press, Milton Keynes.

Hall, S. (1990) Cultural identity and diaspora, in *Identity: Community, Culture and Difference* (ed. J. Rutherford), Lawrence & Wishart, London.

Herman, N.J. (1993) Return to sender: reintegrative stigma management strategies of ex-psychiatric patients. *Journal of Contemporary Ethnography*, **22**, 295–330.

Herman, N. and Musolf, G.R. (1998) Resistance among ex-psychiatric patients: expressive and instrumental rituals. *Journal of Contemporary Ethnography*, **26**(4), 426–49.

Hewison, A. (1993) The language of labour: an examination of the discourses of childbirth. *Midwifery*, 9, 225–34.

Hinshelwood, R.D. (1987) *What Happens in Groups*, Free Association Books, London.

Holbrook, T.L. (1995) Finding subjugated knowledge: personal document research. *Social Work*, 40(6), 746–51.

Holliday, M.E. and Parker, D.L. (1997) Florence Nightingale, feminism and nursing. *Journal of Advanced Nursing*, 26, 483–8.

Hopton, J. (1997) Towards a critical theory of mental health nursing. *Journal of Advanced Nursing*, 25, 492–500.

Jenkins, H. (1988) 'Star Trek': re-run, re-read, re-written: fan writing as textual poaching. *Critical Studies in Mass Communication*, 5, 85–107.

Jylha, M. (1994) Self rated health revisited: exploring survey interview episodes with elderly respondents. *Social Science and Medicine*, 39(7), 983–90.

Kenny, T. (1990) Erosion of individuality in elderly people in hospital – an alternative approach. *Journal of Advanced Nursing*, 15, 1389–401.

Kirsch, G. (1990) Experienced writers' sense of audience and authority: three case studies. *A Sense of Audience in Written Communication Written Communication Annual: An International Survey of Research and Theory*, vol. 5 (eds G. Kirsch and D.H. Roen), Sage, London, pp. 216–30.

Kirsch, G. and Roen, D.H. (eds) (1990) *A Sense of Audience in Written Communication, Written Communication Annual: An International Survey of Research and Theory*, vol. 5, Sage, London.

Kitzinger, S. (1988) Why women need midwives, in *The Midwife Challenge* (ed. S. Kitzinger), Pandora, London.

Jenkins, H. (1988) 'Star Trek': re-run, re-read, re-written: fan writing as textual poaching. *Critical Studies in Mass Communication*, 5, 85–107.

Lakoff, R.T. (1990) *Talking Power: The Politics of Language in Our Lives*, Basic Books, New York.

Long, E. (1994) Textual interpretation as collective action, in *Viewing, Reading, Listening: Audiences and Cultural Reception* (eds J. Cruz and J. Lewis), Westview Press, Boulder, pp. 181–211.

Long, R.C. (1990) The writer's audience: fact or fiction? in *A Sense of Audience in Written Communication, Written Communication Annual: An International Survey of Research and Theory*, vol. 5 (eds G. Kirsch. and D.H. Roen) Sage, London, pp. 73–84.

McQuail, D. (1992) *Mass Communication Theory*, 2nd edn, Sage, Newbury Park, CA.

McQuail, D. and Windahl, S. (1993) *Communication Models for the Study of Mass Communication*, Longman, London.

Mangelsdorf, K., Roen, D.H. and Taylor, V. (1990) ESL students' use of audience, in *A Sense of Audience in Written Communication. Written Communication Annual: An International Survey of Research and Theory*, vol. 5 (eds G. Kirsch and D.H. Roen), Sage, London, pp 231–47.

Marcuse, H. (1964) *One Dimensional Man*, Routledge, London.

Martin, E. (1987) *The Woman in the Body*, Open University Press, Milton Keynes.

Martin, J.P. (1984) *Hospitals in Trouble*, Blackwell, Oxford.

Meehan, E.R. (1990) Why we don't count. In *Logics of Television: Essays in Cultural Criticism* (ed. P. Mellencamp), University of Indiana Press, Indianapolis.

Menzies Lyth, I. (1988) The functioning of social systems as a defence against anxiety, in *Containing Anxiety in Institutions: Selected Essays*, vol. 1, Free Association Books, London.

Ministry of Health (1968) *Psychiatric Nursing Today and Tomorrow*, HMSO, London.

Moores, S. (1993) *Interpreting Audiences: The Ethnography of Media Consumption*, Sage, London.

Morgan, R. and Thomas, K. (1996) A psychodynamic perspective on group processes, in *Identities, Groups and Social Issues* (ed. M. Wetherell), Open University in association with Sage, London.

Mulvey, E.P., Geller, J.L. and Roth, L.H. (1987) The promise and peril of involuntary outpatient commitment. *American Psychologist*, **46**, 571–84.

Park, D. (1982) The meanings of audience. *College English*, **44**, 247–57.

Parker, I. (1992) *Discourse Dynamics: Critical Analysis for Social and Individual Psychology*, Routledge, London.

Pridham, K.F. and Schutz, M.E. (1985) Rationale for a language for naming problems from a nursing perspective. *Image: The Journal of Nursing Scholarship*, **17**(4), 122–7.

Radway, J. (1984) *Reading the Romance: Feminism and the Representation of Women in Popular Culture*, University of North Carolina Press, Chapel Hill.

Russell, D. (1997) An oral history project in mental health nursing. *Journal of Advanced Nursing*, **26**, 489–95.

Ryan E.B., Meredith, S.D. and Shantz, G.B. (1994) Evaluative perceptions of patronising speech addressed to institutionalised elders in contrasting conversational contexts. *Canadian Journal on Ageing*, **13**(2), 236–48.

Said, E. (1993) *Culture and Imperialism: The World, the Text and the Critic*, Chatto & Windus, London.

Samson, C. (1995) The fracturing of medical dominance in British psychiatry? *Sociology of Health and Illness*, **17**(2), 245–68.

Sarangi, S. and Slembrouck, S. (1996) *Language, Bureaucracy and Social Control*, Addison Wesley Longman, London.

Schramm, W. (1954) How communication works, in *The Processes and Effects of Mass Communication* (ed. W. Schramm), University of Illinois Press, Urbana.

Schutz, A. (1972) *The Phenomenology of the Social World*, Heinemann, London.

Scott, C. (1993) *The Influence of Music on History and Morals: A Vindication of Plato*, Rider & Co., London.

Shannon, C. and Weaver, W. (1949) *The Mathematical Theory of Communication*, University of Illinois Press, Urbana.

Szasz, T (1961) *The Myth of Mental Illness: Foundations of a Theory of Personal Conduct*, Hoeber-Harper, New York.

Tajfel, H. and Turner, J. (1979) An integrative theory of intergroup conflict, in *The Social Psychology of Intergroup Relations* (eds G.W. Austin and S. Worchel), Brooks & Cole, Monterey, CA.

Tannen, D. (1989) *Talking Voices: Reception, Dialogue and Imagery in Conversational Discourse*, Cambridge University Press, Cambridge.

Tomlinson, B. (1990) One may be wrong: negotiating with non-fictional readers. *A Sense of Audience in Written Communication. Written Communication Annual: An International Survey of Research and Theory*, vol. 5 (eds G. Kirsch and D.H. Roen), Sage, London, pp. 85–98.

Audience

Valentine, P.E.B. (1996) Nursing: a ghettoised profession relegated to women's sphere. *International Journal of Nursing Studies*, 33(1), 98–106.

Wahl, H. (1991) Dependence in the elderly from an international point of view: verbal and observational data. *Psychology and Aging*, 6, 238–46.

Weissman, J. and Appleton, K. (1995) The therapeutic aspects of acceptance. *Perspectives in Psychiatric Care*, 31(1), 19–23.

Willard, T. and Brown, S.C. (1990) The one and many: a brief history of the distinction. *A Sense of Audience in Written Communication, Written Communication Annual: An International Survey of Research and Theory*, vol. 5 (eds G. Kirsch and D.H. Roen), Sage, London, pp. 40–57.

Wodak, R. (1996) *Disorders of Discourse*, Addison Wesley Longman, London.

KEY REFERENCES

O'Brien, M. (1994) The managed heart revisited: Health and social control. *Sociological Review*, 42(3), 393–413.

Robillard, A.B. (1996) Anger in the social order. *Body and Society*, 2(1), 17–30.

Scheid-Cook, T.L. (1993) Controllers and controlled: An analysis of participant constructions of outpatient commitment. *Sociology of Health and Illness*, 15(2), 179–98.

Svensson, R. (1996) The interplay between doctors and nurses – a negotiated order perspective. *Sociology of Health and Illness*, 18(3), 379–98.

Traynor, M. (1996) A literary approach to managerial discourse after the NHS reforms. *Sociology of Health and Illness*, 18(3), 315–40.

6 TEXTUAL EFFECTS: WHAT DOES TELLING DO?

AIMS

This chapter is concerned with the effects of storytelling in health care. The process of keeping records in nursing and medicine is like writing biographies. Thus, insights from the study of literature can be applied to health care storytelling in order to understand how stories about the lives of patients or clients can so easily become fictional. This fictionality of life histories, preserved in files, may have negative consequences for individuals using health care services.

The disadvantaged position of people from ethnic minorities can be understood from a linguistic perspective. Health professionals' frames of reference to understand human diversity and distress are strongly conditioned along racial lines.

In the case of elderly people, the speech of nurses, and indeed other carers, may be over-accommodated or involve secondary baby talk. This may contribute to the incapacity of the elderly person. Even when communication is not patronizing, misunderstandings occur which could be prevented by more careful choice of words on the part of the nurse.

Participation in the storytelling field defines people's role as patients or nurses. The interchange of stories between patients and nurses facilitates the alignment between them.

INTRODUCTION: LANGUAGE EFFECTS

It is not difficult to identify the overt purpose of all the story-telling that goes on in health care. The official version is that it is there to facilitate care, to enable staff to act in the patients' or clients' best interests and to forestall problems arising from incomplete knowledge. Yet, at its worst, the telling of stories in health care contexts can have a particularly pernicious effect on those who have stories told about them. We have already coined the term 'linguistic entrapment' to describe the possible consequences of health care stories for the client. The inherent ambiguity of human distress and deviance is fixed and controlled through language. Information collected and collated about clients facilitates their management along officially sanctioned pathways of care. As multiple retellings of the client are accomplished, a fictional distance opens up between the client and the corporate biography thus created.

Often we do not know the effects of our language. The literature on misunderstanding and repair suggests that there are many ways in which we routinely renegotiate the meaning of others' talk. Given this indeterminacy, the question of responsibility, of the ethics of language, is particularly problematic.

LITERARY FICTIONS AND LINGUISTIC ENTRAPMENT

The acquisition of a technical language is frequently seen by health care professionals as an important step in becoming an 'insider'. An 'insider', states Tajfel (1982), is one who is familiar with the cultural mores of a particular group. Being able to use a range of technical terms and engage in scientific discourse about patients, clients and relatives is regarded as a sign that professionals have access to esoteric knowledge. The assumption on the part of nursing educationalists is that, if nurses acquire and utilize the discipline's terminologies for verbal and written discourse, they will have an understanding of the meanings embedded in certain words and ideas.

Nurses acquire a technical language as early as their first clinical placement, both as a coping mechanism in an unfamiliar world and as a means of giving the appearance to their senior colleagues that they are more competent then they actually are (Kahn, Steeves and Benoliel, 1994). The language of nursing which has to produce accounts of patients has three cultural sources. The first of these is the language that students encounter in basic training, which is mainly used by teachers and found in textbooks. The second is the language used by practising clinical nurses and the third is the language used in the wider western culture. Kahn, Steeves and Benoliel's study identified that there was no unifying theory of meaning utilized by nurses to represent patients and their problems.

LANGUAGE AS COMMUNICATION OR LANGUAGE AS POWER?

As well as the ostensible functions of language to describe and communicate, the technical language of nursing may also serve to consolidate the power of professionals over their patients. In so far as the vocabulary of nursing is the standard form of language in the health care setting, deviations from this standard by patients can place them at a disadvantage (Ng and Bradac, 1993). Moreover, having a rich and diverse lexicon (as health care professionals do) denotes power (Bradac and Wisegarver, 1984), particularly if it is richer and more diverse than the patient's. Some attempts have been made to describe the effect of diagnostic labelling on patients (e.g. Scheff, 1966) but these were relatively easy for sceptics to dismiss (Kimble, Garmezy and Zigler, 1980). A more thorough examination of language, reasoning, interaction and record keeping in all fields of health care is required.

MAKING SENSE OF SYMPTOMS

Just as nurses need to construct their worlds in terms of the particular paradigm of care that is being used (Garro, 1994), so too do patients.

Previous authors have tended to reduce the therapist's practice to a set of techniques, a list of moral imperatives or to the bland rhetoric mocked by Saleebey (1994): 'Armed with theory and technique, heroically maintaining interpersonal distance and dispassionate concern as he blandishes a variety of esoteric techniques and a precious lexicon' (p. 354).

What is needed is a more nuanced account which sees therapeutic language as a way of constituting the patient and the regime of care, and as a potentially controlling medium (Ng and Bradac, 1993). In therapeutic discourse, Labov and Fanshel (1977) refer to challenges in conversation. Challenges are 'Any reference (either by direct reference or more indirect reference) to a situation which if true, would lower the status of the other person' (p. 64).

The challenge may be overt or buried in requests or statements about events. Making a diagnosis challenges the client who has described his or her symptoms by implying that the symptoms can be accounted for in medical or nursing terminologies. To reconceptualize a reluctance to go shopping on one's own as agoraphobia is to perform a shift that is potentially empowering for the therapist. Crow (1983) describes this as a topic-shading device which accomplishes a linkage between professional vocabulary and what the therapist implies has been present in the client's talk. We have seen this process at work in some detail with Maynard's discussion of the delivery of diagnostic news in chapter 4. Topic-shading devices also function to reduce the uncertainty inherent in the future of the conversation (Berger and Bradac, 1982), enabling some alternatives and interpretations to be preferred over others. The use of topic-shading devices by therapists allows them to impose what linguists call a preference structure. That is, a particular utterance on the part of the therapist implies that certain kinds of answer from the client would be preferred – in general, agreements and positive responses as opposed to negative ones. In everyday talk, when we disrupt the preference structure we often do this by expressing things indirectly and giving an account of why the response is not of the preferred kind (Heritage, 1988). In fact, it's much easier to agree. In nursing, medicine or psychotherapy, it's also much easier for the client to agree with the professional.

In order to guard against professional language glossing over patients' narratives, there are two essential characteristics of being human that health care professionals need to bear constantly in mind:

(1) **Human beings build themselves into the world by creating their own meanings.**
(2) **Culture gives meaning to action by appealing to an interpretive system.**

(Saleebey, 1994, p. 351)

In clinical practice, meanings of the world intersect. The health worker's theories, the patient's story and the myths, rituals and themes of culture all converge in the linguistic interaction. Acknowledging this enables the health care worker not to pathologize or psychologize problems that might better be conceptualized in political or social terms. Until recently, much of the work of practitioners has failed to:

(1) establish a link between individual constructions and the larger environment of social institutions and culture;
(2) examine how any theory of professional practice is also a symbolic construction or 'story'.

(Saleebey 1994, p. 351)

Key reference

With regard to the second point, it is important to note that even scientific accounts of illness have a metaphorical quality (Sontag, 1979) and many scholars now follow the lead of Jacques Derrida (e.g. 1976) in stating that scientific texts exert their effects through their literary style.

Without an understanding of how language can be used to subjugate patients and their accounts of the world, health care professionals' use of language may be inappropriate and damaging. Balint (1957) came to the conclusion that 'By far the most frequently used drug in general practice was the doctor . . . it was not only the bottle of medicine or the box of pills that mattered but the way the doctor gave them to his patient – in fact the whole atmosphere in which the drug was given and taken' (p. 1). Freire (1973) urged professionals who are largely dependent on language for the delivery of their service to:

(1) promote full awareness of the oppressive effects of the dominative knowledge-power institutions;
(2) promote the resurrection to consciousness of local knowledge so that it can be acted upon and used to confront those who would oppress us.

PERSPECTIVES ON MEDICAL LANGUAGE USE

To begin to understand the professional construction of illness, it is worth considering the work done by the medical profession to establish the concreteness of diagnostic categories. Aubrey Lewis's classic work on the concept of paranoia (Lewis, 1970) is critically examined by Harper (1994), who argues that Lewis 'Depicts the history of paranoia as continuous, scientific, coherent and empirically optimistic' (p. 89).

Harper notes how Lewis selects different historical accounts of paranoia and smoothes out the particular idiosyncrasies of the authors who provided them. This method allows the scientific project of psychiatry to establish the constancy and concreteness of the phenomena it studies. Lewis's construction of psychiatry condenses the diversity of accounts of paranoia into a 'Dominant and essentialist view of history' (Harper, 1994, p. 97). That is, he takes the view that there is a single, self-evident truth at the core of every account.

A similar search for truth inspires health professionals to collect information about patients. Lewis's dominant essentialist view of history drives doctors and nurses to assume that a single set of events underpins the incomplete and sometimes conflicting accounts that are the raw material of their work. Chapter 2 demonstrated how textbook authors presume that an underlying reality makes sense of all the conflicting language of health care (Ekdawi and Conning, 1994). Contradiction is problematic and is explicitly avoided by acts of meaning (Bruner, 1990).

In the 1960s, labelling theory (Scheff 1966) was one of the major perspectives on the study of deviance and was welcomed by authors who saw psychiatry as beset with inequalities and dominated by a social control agenda. The theory of labelling encourages us to examine nursing and medical reports as repositories of fiction. Professionals acting as corporate biographers add fictional representations of patients to cumulative records, and may render ineffective therapeutic interventions based on such records. The flesh and blood patient is lost and replaced by a fictional character.

Written text is often regarded as more authoritative than the spoken word, and inaccurate, damaging representations may influence an individual's treatment and even affect their liberty (Goody, 1977; Brown and Yule, 1983; Montgomery, 1986). Written text is transactional rather than interactional (Stubbs, 1980) and relatively permanent. The linguistic straitjacket of medico-nursing reports needs to be acknowledged and countered. The fictionalization of an individual occurs in four important ways.

Firstly, the notion of self is a fluid one. As Olney (1980) states, 'Phenomenologists and existentialists have joined hands with depth psychologists in stressing an idea of self that defines itself from moment to moment amid the buzz and confusion of the external world and as security against the outside whirl' (pp. 23–4). If this is the case, we are forced, like Geoffrey Braithwaite in Julian Barnes's novel *Flaubert's Parrot*, to demand violently: 'How can we know anybody?' (Barnes, 1984, p. 155). Furthermore, an individual's account of himself or herself is problematic. Conway (1990) highlights the reconstructive nature of autobiographical memory and asks, 'How wrong can an autobiographical memory be before we conclude that it is a fantasy?' (p. 2). He demonstrates that autobiographical memory is not a photocopy of our past experience. Disturbingly, it appears to recreate or fictionalize experiences or even wipe them from our consciousness. It may be that the self's life narrative is reconstituted from moment to moment. Autobiographical memories, Conway insists, 'Will never be wholly veridical but rather will (usually) be compatible with the beliefs and understanding of the rememberer and preserve only some of the main details of experienced events' (p. 11).

Even Conway, however, seems reluctant to abandon altogether the notion that there is some sort of essential self underlying autobiographical memory. In psychology, the idea of a self as something that can indeed be represented, for example in a corporate biography (de Man, 1984, p. 71), has been extremely persuasive.

Secondly, human activity takes place in dialogue. Some authors (e.g. Middleton and Edwards, 1990; Edwards and Potter, 1992) have recently scrutinized these largely unexamined psychological models and have reconceptualized memories as the collective creation of particular social situations. This suggests that the process of diagnostic encounters where patients perform their stories for clinicians is an unruly, 'dialogical' activity (Bakhtin, 1984) which makes it difficult to extract a transparent account of the patient. Writing such a transparent account in the patient's records is an activity that we might characterize as monological.

Our memories are what we make them. This argument must be taken very seriously by anyone involved in clinical practice or research. Because we invent or fictionalize ourselves, Olney (1980) is right to highlight 'An anxiety about the self, an anxiety about the dimness and vulnerability of that entity that no one has ever seen or touched or tasted' (p. 23). Like the film-maker Bunuel, we can only speak of autobiographical memory as 'wholly mine – with my affirmations, my hesitations, my repetitions and lapses, my truth and my lies' (Conway, 1990, p. 10). Like the English Romantic poet, John Clare, we might consider biography to be a total 'pack of lies' (Foss and Trick, 1989).

Thirdly, biographies are more rhetorical than 'real'. When autobiographical accounts are made into corporate biographies, fictional distance is significantly increased. In the written record, the patient becomes a constructed representation of the flesh and blood individual. A double fiction operates: the fictional representation of past events in autobiographical memory and the fiction of such representations constructed as text. As Elbaz (1988) indicates, 'Through the processes of mediation (by linguistic reality) and suspension (due to the text's lack of finality and completion), autobiography can only be a fiction. Indeed autobiography is fiction and fiction is autobiography: both are narrative arrangements of reality' (p. 1).

The same argument applies to biography. Representations of an individual biographee by multiple biographers, amounting to a corporate biography, are necessarily an amalgam of narrative arrangements of reality.

Literary critics have proposed that the importance of life writing is 'not that it reveals reliable self-knowledge – it does not – but that it demonstrates in a striking way the impossibility of closure and of totalization (that is, the impossibility of coming into being) of all textual systems made up of tropological substitutions' (de Man, 1984, p. 71). Where a figurative medium such as language is used, there is an inevitable inability to characterize something exhaustively in terms of what de Man calls a totalization. Taking up the ideas of Jacques Derrida, Michel Foucault, Roland Barthes and Jacques Lacan, Olney (1980) states that the autobiographical text

> Takes on a life of its own, and the self that was not really in existence in the beginning is in the end merely a matter of text and has nothing whatever to do with an authorising author. The self, then, is a fiction and so is the life, and behind the text of an autobiography lies the text of an 'autobiography': all that is left

are characters on a page, and they can be 'deconstructed' to demonstrate the shadowiness of even their existence. Having dissolved the self into text and then out of text into thin air, several critics . . . have announced the end of autobiography. (p. 22)

What corporate biographies achieve is the construction of an individual that 'deprives and disfigures to the precise extent that it restores' (de Man, 1984, pp. 80–1). Jaques Derrida suggests that there is nothing beyond the text. Certainly it is difficult to exist as a patient outside health professional routines and storytelling which are an amalgam of perspectives, judgements, opinions and embellishments regarding a patient's life and experiences funnelled into a narrative which replaces the real flesh and blood person.

People's own accounts of themselves may well be ambiguous or contradictory. In effect, they may be asking the fundamental question – Who am I? Again, writings by scholars of literature offer some insights. Sontag (1982) notes how Barthes's autobiography is a book of the dismantling of his own authority or what Thody (1977) has called an anti-biography. For Barthes, 'Who speaks is not who writes, and who writes is not who is' (Sontag, 1982). The biographee, the subject of the biographer, cannot be reduced to a textual representation. People contain tensions, ambivalence and dissonance which are impossible to capture in a unitary, authoritative text.

A further complication to the constructed narrative of patients is added when their records are read. Reader reception theories are concerned with the nature of people's varying interpretations of the same text (Ingarden, 1973; Iser, 1974, 1978; Fish, 1980; Eco, 1981). Readers of any medico-nursing biography will interpret the text in different ways. The fictional character caught in the text will fragment into multiple fictional personalities owing to the interpretative activities of individual readers. In addition, readers have a network of cultural understandings which constitute a literacy within that particular medium (Buckingham, 1993a, 1993b).

Finally, the patient's story is retold: medico-nursing records resemble campfire tales. Fictional distance is at its greatest when readers – from any health discipline – retell the story of a patient to themselves or others. These reconstructions and reverbalizations can result in flesh and blood patients receiving interventions directed at a personality quite unrelated to them – their shadow biographees.

It is clearly naïve to view corporate medico-nursing biographies as transparent representations of individuals although patients' files are often considered authoritative biographies, not fictions. It may be that patients get better in spite of what is written about them rather than because of it. Fictional representations may incarcerate the patient, compromise their liberty or subject them to deleterious identification and stigmatization. Patients who gain access to their medico-nursing biographies may feel like the protagonist in Winterson's *Sexing the Cherry* (1990): 'I discovered that my own life was written invisibly, was squashed between the facts, was flying without me' (p. 10).

RECORDS AS FICTIONS: TWO EXAMPLES

On the basis of an entry in a patient's file notes at a Midlands' hospital, a patient was asked if he had any contact with his two sons. He replied that he only had a daughter. This was ratified on further enquiry. Even at the most factual level, errors occur in the records. Such events fuel concerns about how inferences and judgements about individuals are made. What about the ideological freight (Althusser, 1971) of the words of corporate biographers when descriptions such as 'promiscuous', 'devious', 'manipulative' or 'antisocial' are used of patients? Ultimately, nurses need to ask themselves how much of the information in corporate biographies is fictional, and to counter uncritical readings of the text. The spoken text may have many advantages over the written text in this regard.

A further example highlights the problematic nature of communications between health professionals. A general practitioner sent a short letter to a CPN (community psychiatric nurse) stating, 'Please see this young prostitute with kids who is inadequate and has a personality problem'. On visiting the client, the CPN was surprised to be met by a well-educated, articulate young woman who invited him into a tastefully decorated home. Her two-year old son was happily playing on the carpet with his toys. After some discussion it emerged that the woman had visited her GP stating that she had recently begun to feel very tired and suspected that her haemoglobin might be low. Her GP was at pains to explore her personal life and values. On learning that her rent was partially paid by a male friend and that she was concerned about not being a good enough mother to her son, the GP interpreted the woman within the context of his own moral framework. In the assessment of the CPN, the woman was not a prostitute or inadequate person but a caring and conscientious parent.

Such examples are more than sloppy record keeping or hasty judgement; they are inevitable in a system where narratives are created about patients and different kinds of interaction with the same person give rise to different kinds of narrative (Smith, 1994). The example cited above brings to the fore issues of gender and the problem that feminist theorists have identified of men interpreting women's lives. Nurses need to be encouraged to examine their own practice from the perspective of how conclusions are arrived at about patients.

Fictional accounts of patients can become so diverse that they appear to fly away from the client in a centrifugal fashion. At the same time, the centrifugality of fictional accounts gives rise to a centripetal entrapment. As the flesh and blood person is flung to one side, he or she is simultaneously reincarnated as a fictional construction. They may, unless the linguistic incarceration itself is treated, be subject to future misinterpretations by professionals. Health care relies upon fictional constructions while demanding objectivity. It must promote sceptical reading of corporate biographies and take steps to reduce fictional distance.

RESISTING LINGUISTIC ENTRAPMENT

In a famous painting, Phillipe Pinel is depicted supervising the unchaining of the inmates at La Bicetre hospital in Paris in 1793. As is the case with many good historical stories, this one is probably fictional. In all likelihood, the man who implemented this more humane approach to the care of the mentally ill was Jean Baptiste Pussin, after Pinel had left to supervise another hospital.

Two hundred years later, what can we offer to patients trapped in linguistic chains? How can corporate biographers be alerted to the problematic nature of their productions? How can fictional distance be countered or minimized?

Although language cannot be dispensed with, some of its negative effects might be reduced if health professionals attended more to spoken rather than to written text, because it is the durability of written information which promotes linguistic incarceration and the preservation of fictional biographies. The flesh and blood individual must be privileged over doubtful biography. We need to focus on the word in what we cited earlier as Ong's 'natural [oral] habitat'. Active scepticism about the content of corporate biographies should be encouraged. Nurses should read against the grain of any text. Their writing should be skeletal – relevant, non-judgemental and unembellished. Where nurses in their role as biographers feel fictional distance has opened up within any text, they should be able to make a written rebuttal of doubtful or ideologically loaded information in the form of annotated rejoinders. This would be to follow the advice of Fine (1994), who suggests that the social sciences need more 'rupturing texts with uppity voices' (p. 75). Asking patients to validate written records might be useful to counter fictional distance and would have profound implications for democratizing health care.

Education in all professional health care disciplines should seek to incorporate linguistic awareness. An understanding of the power of language, its ideological freight and the consequences of the written text appearing authoritative is essential for health care professionals and especially nurses, who need to resist naïve presumptions about transparent, scientific language. If nurses recognize that their knowledge of patients is informed by the gender, race, class and sexuality of those who write about them, they are in a position to prevent the records overlaying the voices of the people who are placed in the role of patients.

The second part of this chapter describes a study reported elsewhere (Richards *et al.*, 1996) which examines the sense-making strategies of a group of students as they get to grips with the world of patients. By way of an introduction to the study, the background to

Key reference

the claim that language and social practice in medicine can entrap the individuals who are entrusted to its care is further explored.

PSYCHIATRY, POWER AND LANGUAGE

Key reference

From nineteenth-century feminists to 1960s anti-psychiatrists to 1990s sceptics (Parker *et al.*, 1995), there has been a strong tradition of scholarship which sees psychiatry as a potent agency of social control (Zola, 1972). Like the judicial system, psychiatry is legitimized by and shelters under the auspices of the state and wields the ultimate power to remove the freedom of those who stray from the agreed norms of society (Littlewood and Lipsedge, 1982; Cochrane and Sashidharan, 1995). Just as there has been growing public recognition of injustices and inequalities in the law, psychiatry also has been accused of bias as evidenced by the overrepresentation of ethnic minorities in institutions for the mentally ill and inconsistencies in the process of care and the treatments prescribed (Burke, 1984; Montsho, 1995).

In psychiatry especially, but also in other health care disciplines such as midwifery, the process of care in the UK is argued by some to be shot through with a Eurocentric bias and is accused of alienating and victimizing groups that it purports to help (Cochrane and Sashidharan 1995, p. 3). From this point of view, the caring professions are granted a powerful legitimacy to distort and override patients' own accounts of their experiences and to act on the supposition that whatever is in their professional interest is in the patients' best interests too.

MEDICAL SCIENCE VERSUS SOCIAL CONSTRUCTION

For centuries, problems of the mind have been discussed and theorized about in terms of some sickness inherent in the sufferer. Emil Kraepelin (1883) suggested that toxins secreted by the body were the cause of schizophrenia, and many other nineteenth-century writers and scientists postulated a biological basis for problems of the mind. At the time, cultural differences in the expression of emotional states had been only crudely addressed. Throughout the twentieth century, the medical model has monopolized the care of the mind in distress. Concepts of disease, sickness, aetiology and deficits have been applied to those whose behaviour could not be understood. Medical science has opened up to psychiatry a conceptual lexicon of systematic investigation, measurability, reliability, rules, principles and general laws (Shotter, 1994).

The ideology of scientific knowledge is ratified by the symbolism of the medical culture which is clearly visible upon entry into hospital (Goffman 1961). The training, skills and legally sanctioned professional registration required to operate as a practitioner in such an environment are confined to a small group who are highly regarded in the negotiated order of the hospital environment. Psychiatry relies upon the interpretations of these practitioners, which often preclude any statement of limitation. As Saleebey (1994) puts it, 'The global truth claims of the proponents of "objective reality" – the dominative truth in the western world – subjugate other knowledges and other systems of meaning' (p. 358).

SOCIAL CONSTRUCTION: CULTURE-DRIVEN NARRATIVES

From a social constructionist perspective, human beings, in their attempt to make sense of any situation or event, access frames of reference that are based not only on their own generalized past experiences but also on a multiplicity of interconnecting social and cultural narratives (Shotter, 1993). Hosking and Morley (1991) state, 'Part of this process [sense making] involves learning various narratives, stories, sagas, or scripts about social life. Whatever the language used, the general point is the same. Narratives, stories, sagas, and scripts make explicit the meanings inherent in the social dramas which they portray' (p. 95). Moreover, culture gives meaning to action by situating it in an interpretive system or repertoire (Potter and Wetherell, 1987). This is evident in psychiatry, where mental illness involves an inability to behave in ways that can be understood within the dominant social/cultural context. Staff create meaning out of patients' behaviour by omitting or adding pieces of information in a way that recollects cultural norms, values and expectations. As Saleebey (1994) states, 'There is a link between individual constructions and the larger environment of social institutions and culture' (p. 351).

In the West, cultural narratives about people from other races may preclude them from having good mental health as defined by psychiatric textbooks (*inter alia* Hinsie and Campbell, 1970) and by society in general. White western society's narrative of young black males views them as anti-social, dangerous, aggressive, law breakers, lazy and so on (Rack, 1982) – which accords with the social narrative of mental illness. Thus it comes as no surprise to learn that young black men are overrepresented in both mental hospitals and prisons (Cochrane and Sashidharan, 1995).

People from ethnic minorities, women and people from poor socio-economic classes are more likely than other groups to be stigmatized by psychiatric labels, forcibly incarcerated under the Mental Health Acts, recipients of electroconvulsive therapy and prescribed medication of high strength and dosage (Cochrane and Sashidharan, 1995).

This viewpoint is supported by the findings of Lewis, Croft-Jefferys and David (1990), who found a significant prevalence of negative racial and gender stereotypes among British psychiatrists. Professionals unwittingly interpret patients in ways that complement society's taken-for-granted attitudes, and that override patients' own realities (Crawford, Nolan and Brown, 1995).

NURSES: CO-AUTHORS OF THE PATIENT'S NARRATIVE

Until recently, the work of nurses has consistently slipped through the net of academic researchers who seek to investigate the problems that occur in nursing practice. In many classical critiques, doctors rather than nurses have been perceived as the people with the most power. Recent studies, however, have underscored the importance of nurses in the construction of narratives about patients (Crawford, Nolan and Brown, 1995; Saleebey, 1994).

On a daily basis, nurses spend much more time with patients than doctors. Patients' behaviour is reported by nurses to other members of staff, and may achieve permanence in the form of written records. This information might then influence decisions made by doctors about the clinical management of patients. Each account provides a foundation upon which subsequent authors build, adding new chapters to and new interpretations of the patient's life. Written records, often lurid with value-laden or contentious interpretations, have a long shelf-life which can influence the patient's career even in the absence of the original author or any independent validation.

Taking the case history is the primary step in the authoring of any new patient, and the very act of inquiry is a prominent feature in medicalizing a patient. Taking the case history often marks the introduction of the patient to the world of institutional care. The typically highly structured nature of assessment interviews restricts the information the patient can provide, thereby repackaging the patient's own narrative. In addition, the practitioner may unwittingly engage in sense making and interpretation in order to fill in the gaps where the patient's recollection has failed. In other words, nurses and other health care professionals may try to harmonize conflicting pieces of information.

LANGUAGE, PROFESSIONAL PRACTICE AND ELITISM

The technical and esoteric vocabulary employed by health care professionals serves not only to consolidate and exemplify their power over patients, but also a linguistic bond among colleagues (Ng and Bradac, 1993). Medical language encompasses the patient's medical life (Bradac and Wisegarver, 1984; Cooper, 1970) and deviates sufficiently from the vocabulary used by the lay-person to place the patient at a disadvantage – unable to challenge or even comprehend the clinical assumptions communicated in this dialect or elite discourse (Van Dijk, 1993).

A study of psychiatric nursing students (Richards *et al.*, 1996) provides some practical examples of this process in action. A class of psychiatric nursing students was asked to respond to a series of hypothetical scenarios. Students were given details of several patients' age, race, sex, problems and how they came to be admitted to hospital. In responding to these scenarios, the student participants appeared to access social and cultural narratives about the ethnic group to which the patient belonged in interpreting and making sense of a given situation. In discussing patients, they reproduced race thinking, common sense (Gramsci, 1971) and cultural assumptions as though gleaning facts from the case scenarios themselves.

Confirming the diagnosis

Some participants were quick to provide a rationale for their judgement, which often embellished the information with which they were originally provided. For example, one student commented on a scenario about a man called Andrew Porter: 'This man would appear to be a manic depressive, as he's always changing moods.' The student's statement that Mr Porter is always changing moods is not supported by information presented in the case history. She makes the statement in order to justify retrospectively her opening diagnosis. This is in accord with evidence from research (Mehan, 1990) which suggests that rather than behavioural indicators leading to a diagnostic label, behaviour is interpreted so that it fits the diagnosis.

Pathologizing the black family

The scenario about Delroy Williams, a young black man, states, 'Staff soon contacted his family who eagerly provided a detailed case history', with the word 'eagerly' perhaps suggesting a desire to help. Yet some students chose either to ignore this piece of information or to interpret it in a hostile fashion: 'His parents don't want to know.' This perception of Delroy's family was common. For example:

I don't think he'll get much support from his family.

But if his parents are heavily involved in his return to the community . . . it is likely to make him more rebellious and agitated which will hamper his progress and lead to further breakdowns.

Students seemed to be accessing social perceptions of the black family as dysfunctional or pathological. Howitt and Owusu-Bempah (1994) argue that racist thinking in the social sciences and political debate have promoted the idea of the defective black family which is supposedly characterized by a matriarchal structure, punitive and irresponsible child-rearing patterns and weak emotional ties (Lawrence, 1983). For example, Lobo (1978) comments, 'West Indian childbearing patterns are known to be able to cripple a child's development in the curiously cold and unmotherly relationship between West Indian mothers and their children' (p. 34).

It is likely that in a clinical situation where staff believed the family would have a negative effect on a patient's progress, family involvement might be surreptitiously discouraged. This vilifying of the black family supports oppressive social narrative constructions of black men (Howitt and Owusu-Bempah, 1994).

None of the students alluded to racism as a possible cause for the distress of Delroy or any other black or Asian patient in the scenarios. This was despite widespread scholarly acknowledgement of the importance of racism in understanding black people's distress (e.g.

Cox, 1986; Rack, 1982; Fanon, 1991; Hemsi, 1967; Hickling, 1992; Wetherell and Potter, 1992).

Violence, aggression and harm to others

Violence and being a *danger to others* were recurring themes in the students' responses concerning Delroy despite there being no evidence to warrant such interpretations in the scenario:

> **Delroy is a danger to himself and the public.**

> **Going to need his behaviour restrained to protect others.**

> **Delroy will need strong medication to reduce his violence.**

The case scenario itself gave only the merest hint that Delroy could be violent. Yet students worked the issue of violence against others into their narrative construction of him. It became an important feature of his character to justify high doses of medication.

Responses to the scenario about Jonathan, a young white student who had committed arson, were quite different:

> **I don't think Jonathan will appreciate being in hospital, it might make him worse.**

> **The arson offence is an indication of the frustration or fear that he feels about his studies.**

> **Jonathan's care plan needs to focus on counselling.**

The majority of the students stressed the importance of finding out how Jonathan feels, how he thinks and why he did what he did. This contrasted with the proposed treatment of Delroy, which included long-term admission, physical restraint, seclusion and high doses of medication. The students' responses bore out the well-documented findings that patients of African-Caribbean origin are more likely to be prescribed stronger doses of medication than their white counterparts even when their symptoms and diagnoses are the same (Littlewood and Lipsedge, 1981, 1982; Littlewood, 1988; McGovern and Cope, 1987). None of the students suggested that there might be any reasons for Delroy's supposedly violent behaviour other than his illness. He is not granted a mind in the same way as his white counterpart. It is as if Delroy is somehow not quite as human as Jonathan, and this is reminiscent of the way that Sanders (1993) writes about the granting of 'limited mindedness' to non-human species.

The responses of the students to these scenarios effectively maintain the social narratives that construct both the hypothetical individuals and the racial groups to which they belong. The results of the study are in accord with Lewis, Croft-Jefferys and David (1990), who found that psychiatrists were likely to judge African-Caribbean cases as more violent than white cases, and with Lewis and Appleby (1988), who found that young black males were readily perceived as a danger to others and were therefore recommended for stringent methods of control.

The attribution of reasons

In attempting to make sense of situations, people formulate reasons and explanations which disclose a great deal about the expectations, frames of reference and cultural narratives accessible to the observer, and also the legitimate opportunity granted to the observer to slot his or her explanation into the dialogue of understanding (Antaki, 1994). The process of explaining things works in two directions. Billig (1992) emphasizes the circularity and kaleidoscopic interconnectedness of explanations. For Billig, the very event that we seek to explain is utilized as an explanation for other events.

In clinical practice, the sense making of health professionals is able to prevail over the patient's own reasoning about his or her actions. This is particularly true of psychiatric patients, who are likely to be perceived as unreasonable and irrational. Professional meanings attributed to the actions of the mentally ill provide reasons for what is seemingly bizarre. Such meanings are likely to reaffirm professionals' own stereotypes and prejudices.

Establishing cause and effect

The interplay of cause and effect can be seen in students' responses to the case study of Delroy mentioned above. All the students suggested that Delroy was ill because of frequent cannabis usage, and that his illness and cultural background explained his obsession with religious delusions. For example, one student wrote, 'I've read that some ethnic minorities with schizophrenia characterise their behaviour by religious behaviour which seems to fit in with Delroy's activities.'

In tentatively demonstrating this multiculturalism, the student is at the same time profoundly complicit with the race thinking that many authors have identified in psychiatry and psychology (Howitt and Owusu-Bempah, 1994). Rack (1982) warns that, even though delusions might be false beliefs, they do not necessarily indicate mental illness unless out of keeping with the individual's normal beliefs and those of the group to which the individual belongs. Delroy's beliefs might well be appropriate in his cultural group (Williams, 1981). The student's understanding of cultural diversities serves to consolidate her overzealous diagnosis rather than to facilitate her appreciation of other people's belief systems.

In the second scenario described above, Jonathan was said to be involved with a religious cult. Many students emphasized the importance of exploring this. For example:

Discuss with him how he came to his beliefs in the occult.

A care plan for this patient should focus on talking through Jonathan's beliefs and how he came to believe in them.

However, none of the students thought Delroy's religious beliefs should be discussed with him. It would seem that in addition to the strangeness of a belief, the person who holds the belief is an important factor in health professionals' assessment of his state of mind.

Jonathan is presumed to be able to explain himself whereas Delroy is not.

Delroy's illness was often attributed to cannabis: 'Delroy is no doubt suffering from schizophrenia brought on by constant use of cannabis.' His seemingly bizarre behaviour is now explained in terms of his cannabis use. Despite little formal evidence to support the belief that cannabis induces psychosis, ganja psychosis has become an increasingly popular way of explaining the behaviour of young black men (Howitt and Owusu-Bempah, 1994; Littlewood and Lipsedge, 1982). Thomas *et al.* (1993) report that existing studies have detected no significant difference in the proportion of African-Caribbeans and Europeans who smoked cannabis in the week prior to admission, and Harvey, Williams and McGuffin (1990) found more cannabis use among whites than blacks. Diagnoses of ganja psychosis are often made without the evidence of blood tests and without even asking the patient whether he or she uses cannabis (Howitt and Owusu-Bempah, 1994). In this way, patients' own stories are excluded from the process of diagnosis.

The common-sense nature of reasons

The reasons brought forward by students to explain Delroy's mental distress are presented almost as a matter of common sense. However, as Shotter (1993) points out, 'What one person knows is taken to be, more or less, the same as what the other knows . . . [but] . . . common sense is far from unitary' (p. 173). This disunity of common sense makes it very problematic. Perhaps, as suggested by Billig *et al.* (1988), everyday thinking is shot through with dilemmas. Whereas students' reasoning about Delroy resembled a naïve pharmacological determinism, a more psychological repertoire of thinking was apparent in responding to another case scenario which concerned Hassan Ali, who had lost his job and suffered the breakdown of his marriage:

> He needs to accept the loss of his job and the breakdown of his marriage have caused his depression.

> Hassan became depressed due to being made redundant and his marriage break-up.

> The loss of his family seems to be causing him much grief.

No student mentioned that Mr Ali could be asked whether he felt his divorce had been the major cause of his depression. Instead, students argued in favour of getting him to come to terms with their own world view and presumably thenceforth to manage his emotions in line with some culturally acceptable structure of feeling (Ang, 1985). They did not consider the possibility that Mr Ali's mental illness might have led to the break-up of his marriage or that the mental illness was caused by the marriage itself and not the divorce.

Hassan Ali and Delroy are not credited with the ability to tell their own stories in an intelligible way or to understand the world for themselves. This contrasts with the interest shown in Jonathan's storying. The reasons students put forward for people's distress became powerful influences over the solutions they subsequently recommended (Antaki, 1994).

Enlisting the family as co-therapists

The need for the family to be a part of the recovery process was often referred to by students and this fits closely with professional interest in care in the community. Enlisting the family in therapy has its roots in the popularization of psychotherapy in the 1950s (Parry and Doan, 1994). It is often considered by clinicians to be a vital ingredient in the process of recovery. The family is also used by professionals to make sense of a patient's behaviour.

Many students mentioned the importance of increasing family awareness of the individual's illness as if they expected members of the family to be or become experts in the distress of the patient. Students rarely considered the possibility that families might be unable to provide ongoing support, or be unwilling to assume the responsibility, or object to the conceptual scheme applied to their relative's distress. Students presumed that support was clearly a function of any family.

The information provided by the family about the patient is informed by the narrative that the family has constructed over a number of years and this may differ from the patient's own account (Stone, 1988). Families may have a vested interest in how the patient is portrayed, aiming to present the perceived dysfunction of the patient as a problem in his mind and not in the family unit. Challenges to the family's story made by the patient might be presented by the family as a sign of paranoia, further supporting the psychiatric diagnosis. Instead of being co-therapists, the family can become co- conspirators in the adulteration and subjugation of the patient's own narrative. There is also the danger that use of the family as co- therapists may compromise the patient's confidentiality (Zimmerman and Dickerson, 1994).

MAKING SENSE OF WHAT TELLING DOES IN PSYCHIATRY: LANGUAGE AS A SITE FOR THE STUDY OF HEALTH CARE ACTIONS AND INEQUALITIES

The aim of this study of sense making by nursing students was to investigate the influence and purpose of wider social and cultural narratives in the textual construction of a patient by professional carers. The analysis of the texts produced by the student nurses corresponded in many respects to the depiction of black people in some academic, medical and popular thinking. Many of the previous studies on racism in psychiatry or medicine appear to work with a model of prejudice which emphasizes intentionality. Our position is rather different. We believe that humans can make sense of situations only by employing various sense-making tools which reflect the society in which every caring discipline practises (Hak, 1992). The limited scope of this study only highlights some of the implicit references that

Key reference

181

practitioners draw upon in the everyday act of narrative production and reproduction. However, it is sufficient to indicate how unreflective judgements and stereotypical reasoning may contribute to the process of institutionalization.

This is not to imply that professionals are intentionally engaging in racial biases. Indeed, the evidence from the study suggests that students were attempting to express their knowledge and awareness of cultural implications in psychiatric care, but in so doing they produced statements that were imbued with generalizations about the particular racial group to which the hypothetical patient belonged – statements that were made respectable by a selective rendering of some academic theories.

It can only be concluded, therefore, that rather than being representations of facts or reality, patients' written records are in an important sense works of fiction bearing, at best, slight resemblance to the true nature of things (Capra, 1983). Not only are case notes masterpieces of compression which are able to transform pieces of information, but they are punctuated by the writers' own expectations and interpretations which are deeply rooted in wider social and cultural narratives (Saleebey 1994). Thus the aim of keeping records on a patient in a scientific manner is to some extent defeated by the human quirks of sense making. An examination of the implicit assumptions contained within the patient-practitioner interaction is important in gaining an understanding of the overrepresentation of ethnic minorities in mental health institutions. There is a need for further study to explore language as an important site at which the social action of institutions can be seen at work.

There is a need to find ways of removing the medico-nursing symbols and esoteric vocabulary that so often obscure narratives about patients from the people who matter most – the patients themselves. With knowledge of their own records, patients can more effectively challenge and contribute to what is written about them. Patients must be able to disrupt and hence validate the stories in which they are the central character. By increasing patients' access to medical notes and inclusion of their points of view in records, racism may be reduced in narratives.

ELDERLY PEOPLE: CONSOLIDATING HELPLESSNESS OR FACILITATING AUTONOMY?

Another area of nursing care where stereotypes and prejudices have been found to be a major force in determining the kind of care offered is care of elderly people. It is argued that 'Inappropriate or mismanaged communication can contribute to psychological and physical decline among the elderly' (Edwards and Noller, 1993, p. 207). The speech style adopted by many carers of this client group is sometimes referred to as 'overaccommodated', that is, it assumes a greater degree of impairment of hearing and comprehension than is usually the case. When people in early or middle adulthood talk to older adults they are apt to use secondary baby talk, involving exaggerated intonation and high pitch (Caporael, Lukaszewski and Culbertson, 1983) which simultaneously conveys nurturance and lack of respect.

Speech accommodation theory has been developed by a number of authors, most notably Ryan *et al.* (1986), to provide a framework for exploring the social and psychological antecedents and consequences of modified speech addressed to older adults (see also Coupland *et al.* 1988). Ryan *et al.* (1986) identified four kinds of accommodation in talk between young and old persons. These were:

(a) *Overaccommodation*, which is observed when speakers modify their speech beyond what is needed for hearers who are perceived – sometimes incorrectly – to have some sensory or physical handicap. This is characterized by overly simplified delivery and carefulness of speech.

(b) *Dependency-related overaccommodation*, which relates to the relationship between the giver and recipient of care, typically in institutional settings. This strategy involves overbearing, patronizing speech with overly directive and regulatory features (Coupland *et al.*, 1988; Lanceley, 1985).

(c) *Intergroup overaccommodation*, which involves modification of one's speech based on the addressee's perceived membership of a social group, in this case, older adults. It draws upon stereotypes of this group as less competent, more forgetful, slower, more dependent and less active (Kite and Johnson, 1988; Kogan 1979; Levin and Levin, 1980; Rubin and Brown, 1975; Ryan and Heaven, 1988; Ryan and Laurie, 1990). This kind of overaccommodation involves characteristics of speech which underestimate the hearer's competence and autonomy, such as slowed speech, simplification of vocabulary and grammar, restricted topic selection, impatience and inattention. Arguably, this is the most pervasive type of overaccommodation, according to Ryan, Bourhis and Knops (1991), and relates to the reduced power and lack of status of elderly people in society.

(d) *Age-related divergence*, in which young speakers convey the desire to dissociate themselves from elderly people by talking 'young', for example by using fast speech or slang, discussing youth- orientated topics and showing lack of interest in elders' contributions (Ryan *et al.*, 1986; Ryan, Bourhis and Knops, 1991).

All these features of overaccommodation contribute to lowered self-esteem in elderly people and a reduction in the satisfaction they obtain from communication. Edwards and Noller (1993) found that such clients are likely to evaluate overaccommodation negatively. They argue that when caring for them any modifications to communication should be based on an assessment of individual needs and preferences, as overaccommodation where it is not needed or wanted can interfere with the nursing process. If care-givers communicate in response to individual needs and preferences, the social stereotypes that give rise to overaccommodation will themselves be undermined (Ryan 1991).

In the study of Ryan, Bourhis and Knops (1991), adult participants read scripts of a conversation between a nurse and a nursing home resident. The care-giver was depicted as using either patronizing speech or a more neutral variant, and the nursing home resident was depicted as either alert or forgetful. In the patronizing speech condition, the script featured controlling language and a parental style previously noted in studies of talk to institutional residents (Kahana and Kiyak, 1984; Lanceley, 1985).

Participants rated the nurse in the patronizing condition who used such terms as 'poor dear' and 'good girl' as significantly less respectful and less nurturant, less competent and benevolent than her counterpart in the neutral condition. In addition, participants inferred that patronizing speech was shrill, loud and produced with exaggerated intonation even though there were no overt cues in the written stimulus materials to suggest this. The recipients of the patronizing style were considered to be more helpless and frustrated than were recipients of the more neutral institutional style. The authors concluded, 'Clearly, speaking to elders in a patronising manner on the basis of their age and dependency leads to unfavourable perceptions of the caregiver' (p. 447).

Elderly people or older adults are not a homogeneous bloc and will vary in terms of whether they resent, accept or desire overaccommodating speech. However, possible consequences for this section of the population who are regularly subject to speech overaccommodation include avoidance of speech situations, increased dependency and displacement of anger on to family members. Or they may come to accept the way they are spoken to (Coupland et al., 1988).

In the study of Ryan and colleagues, the fact that patronizing discourse was perceived as less nurturant than the more neutral comparison is at odds with the usual assumption that secondary baby talk is nurturant (Caporael, 1981; Caporael, Lukaszewski and Culbertson, 1983). It may be that nurturance, when administered inappropriately, is seen as insulting.

There is a great deal of research still to be done on speech directed to elderly people. For example, is speech that contains terms of endearment familiar to the hearer patronizing? In the East Midlands of England, the term 'me duck' is commonly used as a friendly term of address, similar to 'mate' or 'dear' in other parts of the country. To a native of Leicester, 'me duck' might pass unnoticed yet be very conspicuous to someone from elsewhere. Research also needs to be done on the gestures and body movements that accompany interactions with elderly people (Lanceley, 1985; McGee and Barker, 1982) and on how they perceive different accents and intonations (Benjamin, 1988; Huntley, Hollien and Shipp, 1987; Stewart and Ryan 1982).

Gibb and O'Brien (1990) conducted a study of the style of speech used by registered nurses in carrying out routine morning care for elderly patients. They began from the premise that conversational interaction constitutes an important part of both the kind of relationship that takes place and its intensity: 'Speech styles associated with routine events in the nursing home context all contribute over time to building an interpretive framework which establishes normative patterns underlying the nursing-home culture' (p. 1389). These normative patterns are 'the constellation of language, activity and social relationships' (Kemmis and McTaggert, 1988) which define that setting. It has long been assumed that nurses develop supportive relationships with clients (Sundeen *et al.*, 1989), yet most discussion of the nursing process emphasizes the techniques for performing tasks rather than verbal interactions.

This prioritizing of technique may lead to activity that is accompanied by minimal or bland conversation with the focus on the nurse getting the job done. Wagnild and Manning (1985) note that task completion is the primary objective so routine procedures are accompanied by stylized conversation. Complex tasks are not likely to facilitate interaction between nurse and client because of the demands the tasks make on the nurse's attention. Gibb (1989), however, found that where procedures are highly mechanical and repetitive, conversation between nurse and resident may be socially rather than task orientated.

The style of speech can change several times in a single conversation. It is polysystemic in nature (Stubbs, 1983). Language is a social activity in its own right (Austin, 1962) and provides an important medium through which to examine patterns of social relations (Turner 1970). Gibb and O'Brien's study (1990) used the notion of speech acts – actions performed through words – introduced first by Austin (1962), then refined by Searle (1979). They assumed that speech acts constitute the basic units of a speech style, so that in a particular style one will find a predominance of speech acts with a particular theme or tenor. For example, there might be more directives to be given during military drill ('Atten-shun!') or more declarations during a wedding ceremony ('I do') than in ordinary social language. In nursing, Gibb and O'Brien argue that the purpose of the physical activity will inform the nature of the speech activity. The interaction occurring within a well-established behavioural sequence may be highly conventionalized (Goffman, 1961) as with the phases of morning care of elderly residents. An excerpt from Gibb and O'Brien's data demonstrates this:

Nurse: All right, you wash your face, dry your face and hands. I'll put your stockings and slippers on while you keep doing your face and hands.
Resident: I did well for Mother's Day.
Nurse: Tell me what you got again?
Resident: I got a shawl, two blouses, slippers.
Nurse: That's good. Now I'm going to put your top on before we stand you up. First of all do a little jump up to release the night-gown. That's a good girl. Now arm first. I'll give your underarms a wash. The towel. Bit of powder? A bit under the arms, there we go. Put

your bra on next. That arm then that arm. Got
everything comfortable? . . . Is A coming today?

Resident: I think so. What day is it today?

Nurse: Thursday. Sometimes she comes on Friday, that's why
I asked . . . We are putting your pink blouse on today.
I like this one. We had better put this on before your
skirt or we will get into a tangle.

(Gibb and O'Brien, 1990, p. 1395)

In this extract, we can see a variety of themes. The nurse and resident discuss Mother's Day, the likelihood of a visitor and what day it is as well as the nurse providing a running commentary and set of instructions relating to the activity in which they are engaged. Conversation is intimately related to the goals of the nursing encounter, as speech act theory suggests. The status of the two people and their role differences are confirmed and consolidated by the nurse's commentary on intimate aspects of self-care. The speech also contributes to the orientation of the client in terms of relating the day of the week to the likelihood of a visit from A.

It is a characteristic of the beginning and end of the human life cycle that other people are allowed to issue a commentary on intimate aspects of the self and the body. In childhood and senior citizenship, toileting, washing and dressing are especially public. They are talked about by care-givers and proficiency at them is rewardable. Even if the talk from the care-giver is not overtly patronizing, there is still a sense that, in having these things discussed at all, one has not yet reached – or has surrendered – an essential aspect of autonomy. Language surrounds us from the cradle to the grave and is intimately connected with the stage in the life cycle we have reached.

MISUNDERSTANDING, MISCOMMUNICATION AND CROSS-PURPOSES: THE DISINTEGRATION AND REPAIR OF COMMUNICATION BETWEEN NURSES AND ELDERLY CLIENTS

Key reference

Van Cott (1993) explored communication patterns between nurses and elderly patients during admission interviews in acute care hospital settings: 'Verbal communication is the primary manner in which patients inform health care providers of their history, symptoms, and concerns and by which health care professionals respond to patients' needs' (p. 184). She found that misperception of speech events represented an important source of conflict in the interactions. Indeed, task-orientated communication often resulted in failure to explore the psychosocial needs of older adults.

Despite the centrality of communication to nursing, from Nightingale to Neuman, the practical emphasis of much nursing activity tends to prioritize physical illness and practical aspects of care. As Van Cott notes, 'Several studies have found that many nurses perceive talking with patients as less important and less effective than the technical aspects of nursing care delivery (Armstrong-Esther and Browne, 1986; Clark, 1985; Faulkner, 1979)' (Van Cott, 1993, pp. 185–6).

Van Cott herself wants to promote a model of the nursing process wherein the quality of nurse–patient communication is important and nurses must be able to communicate with patients in ways that promote trust and encourage disclosure of all relevant problems. She subjected her data to an analysis guided by the communicative competence model of Cassell, Skopek, and Fraser (1976). This model deals with six sociolinguistic variables: (a) acoustics, (b) phonology and syntax, (c) lexicon, (d) conceptions, (e) intent and (f) credence. Van Cott set out to look at miscommunication in these areas.

Acoustics

Acoustical problems such as noise from televisions, other patients' visitors and background hospital noises sometimes resulted in the elderly patient giving misleading information to the nurse. Correcting this depended on the nurse recognizing that the elderly patient had not heard or correctly interpreted the question. Otherwise, miscommunication resulted, leading to inaccurate documentation in the elderly patient's records. Here is an example of one such potentially problematic interchange:

Nurse:	Have you ever had a stroke?
Patient:	A what?
Nurse:	Have you ever had a stroke?
Patient:	Nn, nn, no . . .
Daughter:	[Many strokes.*
Nurse:	Okay, has she ever been hospitalised?
Patient:	[Not that I, not that I know of,
Nurse:	Because of the strokes?
Patient:	No.
Daughter:	Yes, once.
Nurse:	Okay.

*Open brackets indicate conversational overlap. Indentations indicate where conversation was interrupted.

(Van Cott, 1993, pp. 191–2)

Here, the elderly patient reported later that she had not properly heard the question put to her. If the patient's daughter had not been present, this error could have had an adverse effect on her subsequent care. In the case of this patient, hearing and visual deficits combined with environmental noise to have a negative effect on the dyad interaction (p. 192). Van Cott noted that the question 'Do you have difficulty with hearing?' was asked only very late in the interviews between nurses and patients even when the patients appeared to have difficulty hearing. The interview schedule did not allow for nurses to adapt the environment to suit their patients' needs at an earlier stage (p. 192).

Phonology and syntax

'This category involves a breakdown with the knowledge of the language itself or how it is being used (problems arising from non-native speakers of the language, dialects not familiar to the hearer, problems of neurological or physiological origin, or complexity causing confusion for the hearer of the message)' (Van Cott, 1993, pp. 192–3). For example:

Nurse: Okay, I need to know what your expectations are out of this, this hospitalisation. What do you expect out of it?

Patient: Well, ah, I ah, I, I expect all that I'm supposed to get. I don't know.

Nurse: You know, up and walk again type of thing? Or . . . Not . . . Do you expect to be up and

Patient: [Beg your pardon?
          [Oh I

Nurse: walking without crutches?

Patient: expect to be walking. If I didn't think I could walk I wouldn't come in here now. I thought you meant, ah, money wise.

Nurse: Oh no.

Patient: [I don't carry anything.

Nurse: No, I meant if you, what you expect to be

Patient: [Oh yeah, I expect, yes

Nurse: doing after that.

Patient: indeed, hun. That's why I've come here to get rid of the pain.

(Van Cott, 1993, p. 193)

In asking questions nurses have to tread a fine line between being so specific as to foreclose the patients' opportunities for telling their story versus being so general, as in this case, as to create misunderstanding. When problems arose with phonology or syntax in Van Cott's study, it was often because the nurse's questions were not specific enough for the patient to be able to answer them clearly. The patients were also confused when the nurse's statement was ambiguous or incomplete. For example:

Nurse: Your, um, I'd just like to explain to you your watch, your ring, your glasses. Do you have teeth? Dentures. Partial, OK.

Patient: [partial   [partial
. . . I don't know about the ring. You'll need to cut it off. Yeah, it won't come

Nurse: [(laughter)

Patient: off.

Nurse: Okay. That's fine. Just don't worry about it. Um, you don't have to pull it off anyway. Just for . . . the hospital's not responsible for the items that you

Patient: [Oh, oh
Nurse: bring with you.
Patient: [Oh, oh, I thought you meant that I had to take
             it off.

(Van Cott, 1993, p. 194)

Here, the nurse did not complete her initial statement. The patient assumed that her personal effects would have to be removed for medical purposes whereas the nurse was concerned that the hospital should not be liable for their loss. The emphasis on efficient use of time encourages nurses to be brief to the point of not asking for important information or preventing the patient from providing it accurately.

Lexicon

Lexicon relates to choice of words and may cause a problem when nurse and patient do not share the same vocabulary, for example when nurses use medical jargon. Patients have particular difficulty with abbreviations or acronyms such as ECG or ICU and specialist terms such as 'special diet', 'skin graft' or 'seizure'. Van Cott illustrated the difficulties that could arise from use of medical terms:

Nurse: Okay. Have you ever had tuberculosis in the past?
Patient: No.
Nurse: Hepatitis?
Patient: No.
Nurse: Any seizures?
Patient: Not a seizure. A tightness in my chest, but I wouldn't
         call it a seizure.

(Van Cott, 1993, p. 197)

Here, the patient and the nurse seem to have different ideas as to what a seizure is. The patient might have known the symptoms the nurse was interested in by other names. The nurse did not attempt to clarify with the patient what she meant by seizure or how he was interpreting the term.

Conceptions

Conceptions combine semantic information with the senders' and receivers' beliefs about the world: 'Conceptions include ideas, symbols, beliefs, associations, and feelings about a particular thing' (Van Cott, 1993, p. 197). Misunderstanding relating to conceptions emerged when the nurse and the elderly patient could not interpret each other's ideas about blood pressure:

Patient: What's that now?
Nurse: Oh, let's see now, in your right arm it's 170 over 100.
Patient: That's high.
Nurse: Yeah, a little bit. Put your arm up.
Patient: Oh, you take – oh, you take both sides of it now?

> Nurse: Yeah, it's ah . . . it's on the admission sheet to take it on both arms. Okay. Ah, it's going to put there, ah . . . it's 160 over 92.
>
> *(Van Cott, 1993, p. 197)*

In this case the elderly patient's saying 'That's high' revealed that he understood his blood pressure was outside the normal range. The nurse did not, however, clarify with the patient the implications for his health of his high blood pressure. Instead, she merely replied, 'Yeah, a little bit', leaving it to the patient to make his own interpretations.

Intent

Problems occur in the area of intent because the reasons underlying a speaker's statement or question have been misapprehended by the hearer of the message. Understanding the intent of what is spoken implies knowledge of the context, social setting, and the relationship of the participants, as well as the speech itself. As Van Cott (1993) says, 'Elderly patients typically had difficulty understanding the nurse's intentions because the nurse failed to cue or offer the patient an explanation of the purpose behind her actions' (p. 200). For example, when a nurse said to a patient that she wanted to 'check out' her leg, the patient did not cooperate with the nurse because she did not understand why the nurse was asking her to move her painful limb. This was interpreted by the nurse as uncooperative behaviour. Fortunately, the patient's daughter intervened to explain why she felt her mother was not cooperating; otherwise the nurse's impression of the patient and the overall plan of nursing care might have been affected. The difficulty that patients have in grasping nurses' intentions results in talking at cross-purposes:

> Nurse: Can you tell me what you've had done?
> Patient: Where do you want me to start?
> Nurse: Um, let's start now and work back.
> Patient: [now or when I was a child? I could do it backwards or forward but I . . .
> Nurse: [I don't need to know the dates, just the operations that you've had done, or that you're going to . . .
> Patient: [I can't tell you the exact dates.
> Nurse: No, I don't need them.
> Patient: Oh, okay.
>
> *(Van Cott, 1993, p. 201)*

Here, the nurse did not clarify at the outset what she wanted the patient to tell her about her operations. Had she done so, there would have been less confusion for the patient and more efficient use of time.

Credence

This refers to the belief that one places in another person's words. One of Van Cott's interviews demonstrated this problem when the patient doubted the nurse's ability to tell him about the preoperative procedures he might expect (pp. 202–3).

TALK AT WORK BETWEEN NURSES AND PATIENTS

Clearly, this six-part model of different types of miscommunication could be applied to other kinds of nurse–patient interaction. In any situation, the interactive negotiation of meaning is often fraught with difficulty and communication breakdowns are common. However, the significance of communication breakdowns in the nursing process can be very great. There are obvious consequences of non-disclosure of medical conditions, allergies and medication, but there are also consequences that are more difficult to measure, such as it taking longer to elicit the information that is needed, frustration on the part of nurses and patients, anxiety, and the possible labelling of the patient as uncooperative. Van Cott concludes, 'The nurses did not consistently analyse the reasons behind elderly patients' statements that did not directly answer their questions. Time constraints together with a lack of effective use of communication skills made it difficult for the nurses to adequately assess the meaning of the patients' statements' (p. 203). The elderly patients in Van Cott's study used an indirect, narrative approach to answering questions and West, Bondy and Hutchinson (1991) advise, 'Rather than dismissing these apparently irrelevant stories, tune into them. They often provide insight to the elder's opinions and concerns' (p. 175).

Studies such as Van Cott's (1993) and Van Servellen's (1988) underscore the importance of nurses' communication skills. Longitudinal studies would be valuable to examine the effects of the admission experience on the care of the patient during hospitalization and after discharge. There is also a need to address the effects of different methods of teaching interpersonal skills in the education and professional development of nurses. Nursing curricula that encourage effective communication strategies and listening skills are vital.

CONCLUSIONS

What is the purpose of nursing records and nursing language? At first, one might answer that they are to communicate about patients, to tell the reader or listener the significant elements of the problem, the kind of care that is being tried and the outcome – or to enable consistency of care from one shift to the next. Professionals in many nations have this kind of approach to medico-nursing records. In the USA, the Joint Commission on Accreditation of Hospitals (JCAH) says that the purpose of records is 'To furnish documentation evidence of the course of the patient's medical evaluation, treatments and change in condition during the hospital stay' (Joint Commission on Accreditation of Hospitals, 1985, p. 87). This is the model of language in nursing practice which most first-year students would recognize. Many authors are increasingly sceptical of this transparent account of language. Gordon and Buresh (1995) see nursing language as seeking 'Intellectual legitimacy in mimicking the opaque language of physicians. In academia or the hospital, this strategy may advance nursing's cause. In the outside world, it's a recipe for making one's work unknowable' (p. 20). These authors are keen for nurses to get away from the arcane language of doctors and to start making sense to lay-people.

It is clear that nursing records often do not contain even the kind of information that is officially sanctioned. In a study of nursing records in a Scandinavian hospital by Ehnfors and Smedby (1993) it was found that two-thirds of the patients' nursing records had no care plan, 90 per cent had no diagnosis, and in a third of cases there was no note of the outcome. Only one-third of the problems identified in the records were accompanied by notes on the patient's progress. Bernick and Richards (1994) indicate that it is usual to find records of confused elderly patients which contain useless comments such as: 'Patient voided, no voiced complaints. Ate lunch well. Resting in bed' (p. 203).

In this context it is worth asking: what does telling do? It is clearly not about communicating the important features of care. It does not enable staff to 'Communicate their actions and the rationale for their clinical activities' (Bernick and Richards, 1994, p. 203). Perhaps telling in the medical and nursing process is a kind of ceremony, the function of which is to leave some areas of care unclarified. As one of the informants in Tapp's study (1990) commented, 'Nothing charted, nothing critiqued' (p. 236).

Moreover, the telling inherent in the charting process is perceived by some nurses to be largely irrelevant to what they do: 'I think charting doesn't reflect what we do. That's probably why a lot of nurses are resistant to it. It isn't reflective of what we do, what we've done for the patient or even what the patient's problem necessarily is' (Tapp, 1990, p. 236). There appears to be a disjuncture between what nurses perceive as the real business of nursing and the process of documentation.

Are nursing records actually read? Despite the exhortations in the literature about the importance of documentation (e.g. Tapp, 1990; Minda and Brundage, 1994; Pieper et al., 1990), there have been some reports that nursing records are not often read (Walker and Selmanoff, 1964). This is not surprising if writing the record is considered irrelevant and does not capture the process well. If the patient is making predictable progress, record writing and reading may seem a waste of time; it is only when the patient is exceptional that the record may be scoured for clues.

Much effort is being put into encouraging nurses to produce fuller, more comprehensive and more legally defensible documentation. After all, in UK and US law, nursing records are legal documents and can be used as evidence in inquiries and litigation. There are dire warnings in the literature that 'Bad charting will make a good nurse look bad'

(Gruber and Gruber, 1990, p. 255). This chapter has argued that telling does much more than simply keep up appearances. It is interwoven with and helps support the entire process of health care.

Telling is a way of controlling nurses and patients. In an account of counselling people who were concerned about their HIV status, Miller and Silverman (1995) note that clients sometimes adopt professional rhetoric. As the authors say, clients are thus disciplining themselves of their own free will: 'The critical issue for the therapists was the clients' willingness and ability to enter a language of troubles and solutions' (p. 744).

Thus, the effect of telling is to constitute the clients as suitable for the process of counselling. The clients are as keen as the therapists to become part of the institution of counselling.

Telling is part of the whole health care situation. It takes place in offices, wards or clients' own homes, under supervision or out of earshot of superiors; in a written report or as an off-the-record aside. Mutterings between doctors at the foot of the patient's bed while he or she strains to hear are just as much part of the institutional regime of language as hours spent in full and frank discussion with the patient. Language partly constitutes these complex interlocking formal and informal spaces.

An example of this interlocking quality can be found in the experience of a man who suffered a scratch to his eye from a piece of sawdust, and was referred to an eye clinic. While there, he was very distressed to overhear the consultant murmur to a colleague, 'He'll go blind in two years anyway.' Subsequently, he regularly sought assurances from his GP and optician about the state of his eyes and it was only when his eyes did not deteriorate after several years that the fateful words ceased to worry him. This example illustrates how informal and speculative remarks can have profound implications for patients' subsequent use of health care facilities. In this case, the formal reassurances about the patient's eyes carried less weight for him than the overheard remark. He had every bit as sophisticated a view of what goes on in health care settings as many analysts, because he worked on the assumption that the real prognosis was what the doctor muttered to his colleagues, and that what he was being told was mere window dressing. To make sense of what language in health care settings means and what it does, we have to acknowledge participants' own analyses of what those settings are about and what goes on there.

SUMMARY

The language used by nurses may have important practical consequences for their clients and for other professionals. By means of their ability to contribute to clients' records, nurses have the ability to entrap clients in a fictional biography which may bear little resemblance to the flesh and blood person on which it is based. This tendency for language to entrap the people nurses care for can be seen most effectively when we consider certain client groups such as ethnic minorities or older adults.

In the case of clients from ethnic minorities, nursing students tend to grant them less opportunity to express themselves, are more wary of possible violence and are more likely to believe that drugs are appropriate. In the case of elderly clients, nurses are likely to act in a way that consolidates and even exaggerates their incapacity rather than enables them to live independently. Thus language reflects and enhances inequalities that exist in broader society. It is vital that nurses are aware of these possibilities so as to be able to challenge them. In this way, instead of communiciating society's prejudices, nurses can genuinely begin to communicate care.

REFERENCES

Althusser, L. (1971) *Lenin and Philosophy and Other Essays* (trans. B. Brewster), New Left Books, London.

Ang, I. (1985) *Watching Dallas: Soap Opera and the Melodramatic Imagination*, Methuen, London.

Antaki, C. (1994) *Explaining and Arguing*, Sage, Thousand Oaks, CA.

Armstrong-Esther, C.A. and Browne, K.D. (1986) The influence of elderly patients' mental impairment on nurse-patient interaction, *Journal of Advanced Nursing*, 11, 379–87.

Austin, J.L. (1962) *How to Do Things with Words*, Clarendon Press, Oxford.

Bakhtin, M.M. (1984) *Problems of Dostoevsky's Poetics*, Manchester University Press, Manchester.

Balint, M. (1957) *The Doctor, His Patient and the Illness*, 2nd edn, Pitman Medical, London.

Barnes, J. (1984) *Flaubert's Parrot*, Picador, London.

Benjamin, B.A. (1988) Changes in speech production and linguistic behaviour with aging, in *Communication Behaviour and Aging: A Sourcebook for Clinicians* (ed. B.B. Shadden), Williams & Wilkins, Baltimore.

Berger, C.R. and Bradac, J. (1982) *Language and Social Knowledge: Uncertainty in Interpersonal Relations*, Arnold, London.

Bernick, L. and Richards, P. (1994) Nursing documentation: a program to promote and sustain improvement. *Journal of Continuing Education in Nursing*, 25(5), 203–8.

Billig, M. (1992) *Talking of the Royal Family*, Routledge, London.

Billig, M., Condor, S., Edwards, D., Gane, M., Middleton, D. and Radley, A. (1988) *Ideological Dilemmas: A Social Psychology of Everyday Thinking*, Sage, London.

Bradac, J.J. and Wisegarver, R. (1984) Ascribed status, lexical diversity and accent: determinants of perceived status, solidarity and control of speech style. *Journal of Language and Social Psychology*, 3, 239–55.

Brown, G. and Yule, G. (1983) *Discourse Analysis*, Cambridge University Press, Cambridge.

Bruner, J. (1990) *Acts of Meaning*, Harvard University Press, Cambridge, MA.

Buckingham, D. (1993a) *Children Talking Television: The Making of Television Literacy*, Falmer, London.

Buckingham, D. (ed.) (1993b) *Reading Audiences: Young People and the Media*, Manchester University Press, Manchester.

Burke, A. (1984) Racism and psychological disturbance among West Indians in Britain. *International Journal of Social Psychiatry*, 30, 50–68.

Capra, F. (1983) *The Turning Point*, Bantam Books, New York.

Caporael, L.R. (1981) The paralanguage of care giving: baby talk to the institutionalised aged. *Journal of Personality and Social Psychology*, **40**(5), 876–884.

Caporael, L.R., Lukaszewski, M.P. and Culbertson, G.H. (1983) Secondary baby talk: judgements by institutionalised elderly and their caregivers. *Journal of Personality and Social Psychology*, **44**(4), 746–54.

Cassell, E.J., Skopek, L. and Fraser, B. (1976) A preliminary model for the examination of doctor–patient communication. *Language Sciences*, (December), 10–13.

Clark, J.M. (1985) The development of research in interpersonal skills in nursing, in *Interpersonal Skills in Nursing: Research and Applications* (ed. C. Kagan), Croom Helm, London.

Cochrane, R. and Sashidharan, S. P. (1995) *Mental Health and Ethnic Minorities: A Review of the Literature and Implications for Services*, University of Birmingham and Northern Birmingham Mental Health Trust, Birmingham.

Conway, M.A. (1990) *Autobiographical Memory: An Introduction*, Open University Press, Milton Keynes.

Cooper, J.E. (1970) The use of a procedure for standardising psychiatric diagnosis, in *Psychiatric Epidemiology* (eds E.H. Hare and J.K. Wing), Oxford University Press, London.

Coupland, N., Coupland, J., Giles, G. and Henwood, K. (1988) Accommodating the elderly: invoking and extending a theory. *Language in Society*, **17**(1), 1–42.

Cox, J.L. (ed.) (1986) *Transcultural Psychiatry*. Croom Helm, London.

Craib, I. (1994) *The Importance of Disappointment*, Routledge, London.

Crawford, P., Nolan, P and Brown, B. (1995) Linguistic entrapment: medico-nursing biographies as fictions. *Journal of Advanced Nursing*, **22**, 1141–8.

Crow, B.K. (1983) Topic shifts in couples' conversations, in *Conversational Coherence: Structure and Strategy* (eds R.T. Craig and K. Tracy), Sage, Beverley Hills, CA, pp. 136–56.

de Man, P. (1984) Autobiography as de-facement, in *The Rhetoric of Romanticism*, Columbia University Press, New York.

Derrida, J. (1976) *Of Grammatology* (Translated by G.C. Spivak), Johns Hopkins Press, Baltimore.

Eco, U. (1981) *The Role of the Reader: Explorations in the Semiotics of Text*, Hutchinson, London.

Edwards, D. and Potter, J. (1992) *Discursive Psychology*, Sage, London.

Edwards, H. and Noller, P. (1993) Perceptions of overaccommodation used by nurses in communication with the elderly. *Journal of Language and Social Psychology*, **12**(3), 207–23.

Ekdawi, M.Y. and Conning, A.M. (1994) *Psychiatric Rehabilitation: A Practical Guide*, Chapman & Hall, London.

Elbaz, R. (1988) *The Changing Nature of Self: A Critical Study of the Autobiographical Discourse*, Croom Helm, London.

Ehnfors, M. and Smedby, B. (1993) Nursing care as documented in patient records. *Scandinavian Journal of Caring Sciences*, 7, 209–20.

Fanon, F. (1991). *Black Skin, White Masks*, 2nd edn, Pluto Press, London.

Faulkner, A. (1979) Monitoring nurse–patient interaction in a ward. *Nursing Times*, **75**(23), 95–6.

Fine, M. (1994) Working the hyphens: reinventing self and other in qualitative research, in *Handbook of Qualitative Research* (eds N. Denzin and Y.S. Lincoln), Sage, Thousand Oaks, CA, pp. 70–82.

Fish, S. (1980) *Is There a Text in This Class? The Authority of Interpretative Communities*, Harvard University Press, Cambridge, MA.

Foss, A. and Trick, K. (1989) *St Andrews Hospital Northampton: The First 150 Years*, Cambridge University Press, Cambridge.

Freire, P. (1973) *Pedagogy of the Oppressed*, Seabury Press, New York.

Garro, L. C. (1994) Narrative representations of chronic illness experiences: cultural models of illness, mind, and body in stories concerning the temporomandibular joint. *Social Science and Medicine*, 38, 775–88.

Gibb, H. (1989) This is what we have to do – are you OK? Nurses' speech with elderly nursing home residents. Unpublished research report, Deakin University, Geelong, Australia.

Gibb, H. and O'Brien B. (1990) Jokes and reassurance are not enough: ways in which nurses relate through conversation with elderly clients. *Journal of Advanced Nursing*, 15, 1389–401.

Gilbert, G.N. and Mulkay, M. (1984) *Opening Pandora's Box: A Sociological Analysis of Scientists' Discourse*, Cambridge University Press, Cambridge.

Goffman, E. (1961) *Asylums*, Doubleday, Garden City, NY.

Goody, J. (1977) *The Domestication to the Savage Mind*, Cambridge University Press, Cambridge.

Gordon, S. and Buresh, B. (1995) Nursing in the right words: to make lay people see and feel what nurses do you have to speak their language. *American Journal of Nursing*, (March), 20–2.

Gramsci, A. (1971) *Selections from the Prison Notebooks*, Lawrence & Wishart, London.

Gruber, M. and Gruber, J.M. (1990) Nursing malpractice: the importance of documentation, or saved by the pen. *Gastroenterology Nursing*, 12(4), 255–9.

Harper, D.J. (1994) Histories of suspicion in a time of conspiracy: a reflection on Aubrey Lewis's history of paranoia. *History of the Human Sciences*, 7(3), 89–109.

Harvey, I., Williams, M. and McGuffin, P. (1990) The functional psychoses of Afro-Caribbeans. *British Journal of Psychiatry*, 157, 515–22.

Hemsi, L.K. (1967) Psychiatric morbidity of West Indian immigrants. *Social Psychiatry*, 2, 95–100.

Heritage, J. (1988) Explanations as accounts: a conversation analytic perspective, in *Analysing Everyday Explanation* (ed. C. Anatki), Sage, London, pp. 95–117.

Hickling, F. (1992) Racism: an Afro-Jamaican perspective. *British Medical Journal*, 305, 1102.

Hinsie, J. and Campbell, R. (1970) *Psychiatric Dictionary*, 4th edn, Oxford University Press, New York.

Hosking, D. and Morley, I. (1991) *A Social Psychology of Organising: People, Processes and Contexts*, Harvester Wheatsheaf, London.

Howitt, D. and Owusu-Bempah, J. (1994) *The Racism of Psychology: Time for a Change*, Harvester Wheatsheaf, London.

Huntley, R., Hollien, H. and Shipp, T. (1987) Influence of listener characteristics on perceived age estimations. *Journal of Voice*, 1, 49–52.

Ingarden, R. (1973) *The Literary Work of Art*, University of Illinois Press, Evanston, IL.

Iser, W. (1974) *The Implied Reader*, Johns Hopkins University Press. Baltimore.

Iser, W. (1978) *The Act of Reading*, Allen Lane, London.

Joint Commission on Accreditation of Hospitals (1985) *Accreditation Manual for Hospitals*, JCAH, Chicago.

Kahana, E. and Kiyak, H.A. (1984) Attitudes and behaviours of staff facilities for the aged. *Research on Aging*, 6, 395–416.

Kahn, D. L., Steeves, R. H. and Benoliel, J. Q. (1994) Nurses' views of the coping of patients. *Social Science and Medicine*, 38, 1423–30.

Kemmis, S. and McTaggert, R. (1988) *The Action Research Planner*, Deakin University Press, Geelong, Victoria.

Kimble, G.A., Garmezy, N. and Zigler, E. (1980) *Principles of General Psychology*, John Wiley, New York.

Kite, M.E. and Johnson, B.T. (1988) Attitudes toward older and younger adults: a meta-analysis. *Psychology and Aging*, 3, 233–44.

Kogan, N. (1979) Beliefs, attitudes and stereotypes about old people. *Research on Aging*, **1**, 11–36.

Kraepelin, E. (1883) *Clinical Psychiatry* (trans. R. Diefendorf), Scholars' Facsimiles and Reprints, Delmar, NY.

Labov, W. and Fanshel, D. (1977) *Therapeutic Discourse: Psychotherapy as Conversation*, Academic Press, New York.

Lanceley, A: (1985) Use of controlling language in rehabilitation of the elderly. *Journal of Advanced Nursing*, **10**, 125–35.

Lawrence, E. (1983) In the abundance of water the fool is thirsty, in *The Empire Strikes Back* (ed. Centre for Contemporary Cultural Studies), Hutchinson, London.

Levin, J. and Levin, W.C. (1980) *Ageism: Prejudice and Discrimination against the Elderly*, Wadsworth, Belmont, CA.

Lewis, A. (1970) Paranoia and paranoid: a historical perspective. *Psychological Medicine*, **1**, 2–12.

Lewis, G. and Appleby, L. (1988) Personality disorder: the patients psychiatrists dislike. *British Journal of Psychiatry*, **153**, 44–9.

Lewis, G., Croft-Jefferys, C. and David, A. (1990) Are British psychiatrists racist? *British Journal of Psychiatry*, **157**, 410–15.

Littlewood, R. and Lipsedge, M. (1981) Some social and phenomenological characteristics of psychotic immigrants. *Psychological Medicine*, **11**, 289–320.

Littlewood, R. and Lipsedge, M (1982) *Aliens and Alienists: Ethnic Minorities and Psychiatry*, Penguin, Harmondsworth.

Littlewood, R. (1988) Community initiated research: a study of psychiatrists' conceptualisations of 'cannabis psychosis'. *Psychiatric Bulletin*, **12**, 486–8.

Lobo, E. (1978) *Children of immigrants to Britain: their health and social problems*. Allen & Unwin, London.

McGee, J. and Barker, M. (1982) Deference and dominance in old age: an exploration of social theory. *International Journal of Aging and Human Development*, **15**, 247–62.

McGovern, D. and Cope, R. (1987) The compulsory detention of males from different ethnic minorities, with special reference to Offender Patients. *British Journal of Psychiatry*, **150**, 505–12.

Mehan, H. (1990) Oracular reasoning in a psychiatric exam: the resolution of conflict in language, in *Conflict Talk: Sociolinguistic Investigations of Arguments in Conversations* (ed. A.D. Grimshaw), Cambridge University Press, Cambridge.

Middleton, D. and Edwards, D. (1990) *Collective Remembering*, Sage, London.

Migliore. S. (1993) 'Nerves': the role of metaphor in the cultural framing of experience. *Journal of Contemporary Ethnography*, **22**(3), 331–60.

Miller, G. and Silverman, D. (1995) Troubles talk and counselling discourse. *Sociological Quarterly*, **36**(4), 725–47.

Minda, S. and Brundage, D.J. (1994) Time differences in hand-written and computer documentation of nursing assessment. *Computers in Nursing*, **12**(6), 277–9.

Montgomery, M. (1986) *An Introduction to Language and Society*, Routledge & Kegan Paul, London.

Montsho, Q. (1995) Behind locked doors, in *Talking Black* (ed. V. Mason-John), Cassell, London.

Mulkay, M. (1985) *The Word and the World: Explorations in the Forms of Sociological Analysis*, Allen Unwin, London.

Ng, S. H. and Bradac, J.J. (1993) *Power in Language: Verbal Communication and Social Influence*, Sage, London.

Olney, J. (1980) Autobiography and the cultural movement: a thematic, historical and bibliographical introduction, in *Autobiography: Essays Theoretical and Critical*, Princeton University Press, Princeton.

Parker, I., Georgaca, E., Harper, D., McLaughlin, T. and Stowell-Smith, M. (1995) *Deconstructing Psychopathology*, Sage, London and Thousand Oaks, CA.

Parry, A. and Doan, R.E. (1994) *Story Re-visions: Narrative Therapy in the Postmodern World*, Guilford Press, London.

Pieper, B., Mikols, C., Mance, B. and Adams, W. (1990) Nurses' documentation about pressure ulcers. *Decubitus*, **3**(1), 32–7.

Potter, J. and Wetherell, M. (1987) *Discourse and Social Psychology: Beyond Attitudes and Behaviour*, Sage, London.

Rack, P. (1982) *Race, Culture and Mental Disorder*, Tavistock Publications, London.

Rennie, D. L (1994) Storytelling in psychotherapy: the client's subjective experience. *Psychotherapy*, **31**(2), 235–43.

Rubin, K.H. and Brown, I.D.R. (1975) A life span look at person perception and its relationship to communicative interaction. *Journal of Gerontology*, **30**, 461–8.

Ryan, E.B. (1991) Attitudes and behaviours toward older adults in communication contexts. Paper presented at the Fourth International Conference on Language and Social Psychology, Santa Barbara, CA, August.

Ryan, E.B., Bourhis, R.Y. and Knops, U. (1991) Evaluative perceptions of patronising speech addressed to elders. *Psychology and Aging*, **6**(3), 442–50.

Ryan, E.B., Giles, H., Bartolucci, G. and Henwood, K. (1986) Psycholinguistic and social psychological components of communication by and with the elderly. *Language and Communication*, **6**, 1–24.

Ryan, E.B. and Heaven, R.K.B. (1988) The impact of situational context on age based attitudes. *Social Behaviour*, **3**, 105–117.

Ryan, E.B. and Laurie, S. (1990) Evaluations of older and younger adult speakers: the influence of communication effectiveness and noise. *Psychology and Aging*, **5**, 514–19.

Saleebey, D. (1994) Culture, theory and narrative: the intersection of meanings in practice. *Social Work*, **39**, 351–9.

Sanders, C. R. (1993) Understanding dogs: caretakers' attribution of mindedness in canine-human relationships. *Journal of Contemporary Ethnography*, **22**(2), 205–26.

Scheff. T. (1966) *Being Mentally Ill: A Sociological Theory*, Aldine, Chicago.

Searle, J. (1979) *Expression and Meaning: Studies in the Theory of Speech Acts*, Cambridge University Press, Cambridge.

Shotter, J. (1993) *The Cultural Politics of Everyday Life*, Open University Press, Milton Keynes.

Shotter, J. (1994) *Conversational Realities: Constructing Life through Language*, Sage, Thousand Oaks, CA.

Smith, L.M. (1994) Biographical method, in *Handbook of Qualitative Research* (eds N. Denzin and Y.S. Lincoln), Sage, Thousand Oaks, CA, pp. 273–85.

Sontag, S. (ed.) (1982) *A Barthes Reader*, Jonathan Cape, London.

Stewart, M.A. and Ryan, E.B. (1982) Attitudes toward younger and older adult speakers: effects of varying speech rates. *Journal of Language and Social Psychology*, **1**, 91–109.

Stone, E. (1988) *Black Sheep and Kissing Cousins*, Penguin, New York.

Stubbs, M. (1980) *Language and Literacy: The Sociolinguistics of Reading and Writing*, Routledge & Kegan Paul, London.

Stubbs, M. (1983) *Discourse Analysis: The Sociolinguistic Analysis of Natural Language*, Blackwell, Oxford.

Sundeen, S.J., Stuart, G.W., DeSalvo-Rankin, E.A. and Cohen, S.A. (1989) *Nurse–client interaction*, 4th edn, Mosby, St Louis.

Tajfel, H. (1982) Social psychology of intergroup relations. *Annual Review of Psychology*, **33**, 1–39.

Tapp, R.A. (1990) Inhibitors and facilitators to documentation of nursing practice. *Western Journal of Nursing Research*, **12**(2), 229–40.

Thody, P. (1977) *Roland Barthes: A Conservative Estimate*, Macmillan, London.

Thomas, C.S., Stone, K., Osborn, M., Thomas, P.F. and Fisher, M. (1993) Psychiatric morbidity and compulsory admission among UK born Europeans, Afro-Caribbeans and Asians in Central Manchester. *British Journal of Psychiatry*, **163**, 91–9.

Turner, R. (1970) Words, utterances and activities, in *Understanding Everyday Life* (ed. J.D. Douglas), Routledge & Kegan Paul, London.

Van Dijk, T.A. (1993) *Elite Discourse and Racism*, Sage, London.

Van Servellen, G. (1988) Nurses' perceptions of individualised care in nursing practice. *Western Journal of Nursing Research*, **10**, 291–301.

Wagnild, G. and Manning, R. (1985) Convey respect during bathing procedures. *Journal of Gerontological Nursing*, **11**(12), 6–10.

Walker, V.H. and Selmanoff, E.D. (1964) A study of the nature and use of nurses' notes. *Nursing Research*, **13**, 113–21.

West, M., Bondy, E. and Hutchinson, S. (1991) Interviewing institutionalised elders: threats to validity. *Image: Journal of Nursing Scholarship*, **23**, 171–6.

Williams, K.M (1981) *The Rastafarians*, Ward Lock Educational, London.

Winterson, J. (1990) *Sexing the Cherry*, Vintage, New York.

Zimmerman, J. and Dickerson, V. (1994) Using a narrative metaphor: implications for theory in clinical practice. *Family Processes*, **33**, 233–67.

KEY REFERENCES

Hak, T. (1992) Psychiatric records as transformations of other texts, in *Text in Context: Contributions to Ethnomethodology* (eds G. Watson and R.M. Seiler), Sage, Newbury Park, CA.

Richards, K.D., Brown, B., Crawford, P. and Nolan, P. (1996) Making sense of patients: an analysis of practical reasoning by psychiatric nursing students. *UCE Studies in Language and Literature*, **2**, 1–23.

Sontag, S. (1979) *Illness as Metaphor*, Allen Lane, London.

Van Cott, M.L. (1993) Communicative competence during nursing admission interviews of elderly patients in acute care settings. *Qualitative Health Research*, **3**(2), 184–208.

Wetherell, M. and Potter, J. (1992) *Mapping the Language of Racism*, Harvester Wheatsheaf, London.

Zola, I.R (1972). Medicine as an institute of social control: the medicalising of society. *Sociological Review*, **20**(4), 487–504.

7 Conclusion: How Can We Tell it Differently? Or, Towards Reflective Heresy

In this final chapter we shall attempt to sum up what has been written so far and offer some further thoughts on the state of language in nursing. It is here that we shall attempt to draw back and grasp some of the broader political developments that enshroud nursing as we approach the millennium and identify the links between these and the language that is used, abused and created in health care settings. Among the many ideas we wish readers to derive from this book is that words and their meanings are not fixed, despite the psychological need people have to believe that they are. We want to encourage nurses to dispel this myth.

As well as drawing together the threads we have unpicked in the previous chapters it is our intention to identify two possible directions for the future of nursing language. The first of these is what we consider to be a nightmarish vision of its regulation and control; the second more benign vision involves a more productive critical reflection upon its diversities and possibilities.

The first thing to do as this book draws to a close is to consider what we have left the reader with. Then, having done this, we shall give readers a little 'escape velocity' from their orbit through our selection of ideas, theories and studies, enabling them to apply these to their working lives.

In chapter 1 we introduced the reader to the significance of the way that nurses tend to describe aspects of their health work. We examined how diverse ideologies are joined by diverse understandings of what is *meant* by nursing, a destabilization that is part of a wider concern about the status of meaning and language which comes under the umbrella of postmodernism. In an atmosphere of competing ideologies and discourses, we suggested the urgency for nurses to monitor and transform health care language and consequently construct a different health care reality. In other words, we believe nurses can modify the experience of care-giving or illness by means of the way they use and receive language. Nurses can fortify their own language to compete, for example, with the market language that has invaded health care provision over recent years. In order to continue in their tradition of patient advocacy, nurses need to pay closer attention to the powerful effects of language. This includes nurses becoming more aware of the stories they tell about patients and the stories patients tell about themselves. We alerted the reader to the concept of language as action and to the potentially harmful effects of nursing communication, not just in terms of what is said or written, but in terms of how what is spoken or written is heard, read, interpreted and responded to. We established our concern that the language of helping may override language that depicts the negative consequences of that help, and that nurses may find themselves using language to the detriment of patients, or 'firing paper bullets' at them. We stated that the language of nursing is at the hub of nursing practice. It is where nursing measurement of fellow human beings truly begins.

We explored issues surrounding authorship or 'who tells' in nursing in chapter 2. We demonstrated that authorship is not the preserve of any individual, but is an amalgamated or corporate event shaped by wider cultural contexts. We noted how what individuals write is crucially informed by the politics, values and prejudices of contemporary society. In other words, broader social relations affect authorship, some of which the individual may not even be conscious of. Postmodern scepticism about authorship replaces the modernist view of individuals as authors of their own ideas, speech and writing. This shift heralds an awareness of the historical, professional and academic background of what nurses say and how they deploy the resources of their professional wisdom upon the raw material of clients' accounts of their troubles. Nurses are part of an interpretive community that uses particular language genres or registers that ensure that therapy appears to be effective. To do this nurses rely heavily on referring to other authorities as sources for statements. In essence, nurses frequently speak other people's lines, not their own. The messy business of nursing is compressed into socially sanctioned rational categories or terminologies. Stories of distress are filtered through professional frames of understanding, interviews and documentation. Such filtering often edits out cultural variations in stories of distress and controls the very producers of documentary accounts. Human distress is cunningly repackaged in the health care environment as much by language as anything else. Illness stories are told in a way that facilitates the health care business. We argue that the drive towards documentational accuracy and completeness can only take us so far. We consider nurses who believe that documentation does not reflect what they do are in some ways quite philosophically sophisticated. Ultimately, nurses are involved in a complex linguistic dance. It is important for them to increase their awareness of who speaks *behind* their speaking, or writes *behind* their writing. By recognizing the generative work involved in authorship nurses may step into a new way of thinking about their profession and gain a new measure of creative control over their contribution to the complex storytelling that goes on in health care settings.

Chapter 3 examined how nurses communicate or tell things. Here we extended the reader's knowledge of the operation of genre and register in the language of nursing speech and writing. We demonstrated how nursing communication has distinctive forms and resembles an 'operating theatre' in which textually mediated realities are constructed and, indeed, reconstructed. We provided an outline of the form of nursing communication in three sections. Firstly, we revealed some generic features of nursing language in our account of how nursing students made sense of 'depression'. This included discussion of the politics of reported speech. Secondly, we outlined both proximal and distal features of record making. Thirdly, we looked at the oral and written media of expression. We called for those involved in nursing education to develop the curriculum to provide for a more sceptical reflexivity regarding language use in nursing. We argued that the key nursing values of assisting patients and relieving suffering are best achieved by a constant vigilance about language.

The status of meaning or what is told in nursing language reflects a wider set of debates about meaning in general. This was dealt with in chapter 4, where we viewed health care environments as factories for packaging distress in ways that can be dealt with and about which a meaningful story can be told. Meaning, and particularly the meaning of nursing work, is central to negotiating identities and stories in the health care workplace. The meanings nurses assign to their work has important political consequences. Images of the self as fearlessly tending the sick may not equip practitioners for changing the circumstances in society which produce that sickness. Indeed, they contribute to encapsulating the meaning of illness as an individuated phenomenon susceptible to individuated solutions. Although meanings in health care can be contested between patients and professionals, often we see the meaning of distress legislated rather than negotiated. Even when it appears that health care clients are negotiating the meaning of their problems autonomously, we must be alert to the possibility that professionals are guiding them and providing the spaces into which their distress can unfold.

In chapter 5 we tackled the issue of audience, or who it is that nursing tells its story to. We established the nature and significance of audience in communication, and the way that nurses have to speak or write to a whole variety of audiences who stand in judgement over them, be they individuals or groups. Nurses can be seen to form a kind of textual community in which collective readings of patients circulate. We highlighted the need for an ethics of listening/reading as much as speaking/writing. Nurses need to listen to and read sceptically the speech and writings of fellow health care professionals of all disciplines. Thus, nurses need to value the power of being an audience themselves, helping to shape what others say or write by their responses to it. In order to stand as true advocates of those in their care, nurses need to grasp fully their responsibilities, not simply as textual producers, but also as textual receivers. If they do not take a principled and vigilant stand among the textual communities of health care, nursing will continue its erstwhile weak role in textual power play. It is also important to keep in mind when considering the question of audiences what is not seen or heard as well as what is.

Finally, we established in chapter 6 some of the detrimental effects of nursing language or what the stories it tells can do. Here we examined the fictionality of patient's files, racism in nursing accounts, and patronizing speech patterns in the nursing care of older people. The tendency for nursing language to entrap patients can be seen most effectively when we consider certain patient groups such as those from ethnic minorities or elderly people. In the case of ethnicity, nursing students tend to grant people from ethnic minorities with suspected mental health problems less opportunity to express themselves and are more wary of possible violence from them and thus advocate greater use of medication. In the case of elderly people, nurses are likely to use language that consolidates and even exaggerates their incapacity rather than enabling them to live independently. Thus language reflects and enhances inequalities that exist in broader society. It is vital that nurses become aware of the powerful and detrimental effects of these and other language actions on those they care for. In this way, rather than communicating society's various prejudices, nurses can genuinely begin to communicate care.

Our central tenet, then, is that language is seldom neutral – it is usually an active force in the social world. We hope to have given the reader a sense of how scholars have attempted to make sense of this, for example by seeing language as a bearer of ideology or as reflecting the multiple, unresolvable stories so beloved of postmodernists. This highlights the importance of paying attention to language in nursing, as the discipline is centrally concerned with talk, writing and record keeping. We have also highlighted patients' narratives of illness, for it is through these storied processes of sense making that we come to experience illness and make sense of it to any health professionals we encounter. How nurses use language to make sense of patients can systematically influence the kinds of questions that get asked and the types of treatments provided. Whether we ask a young woman with abdominal pains about contraceptive practices, for example, may well depend on what ethnic group she happens to belong to.

Language is important also from the point of view of telling the story of helping. Medical or psychiatric treatments may appear painful or humiliating – it is through language that they are reframed as something beneficial. Sometimes it is as if the theoretical models of care take precedence over the flesh and blood patients to whom they are directed. This conclusion, therefore, should reaffirm the emphasis that nurses need to be alert to how language is used to construct truths or portray the world in a favourable light. It is only by being aware in this way that nurses can safeguard their patients' interests and those of their profession.

DEFINING NURSING FOR THE FUTURE: STATIC DESCRIPTIONS AND DYNAMIC PROCESSES

There is a danger in attempting to describe language as if it were something that could be fixed and measured. If we count the words or analyse the sentence structure, we will never be able to characterize fully the business of nursing. Understanding the language used at work involves a great deal more than checking the words in a dictionary. Nursing and the language it uses have arisen out of a complex interplay of social forces. A number of interest groups, including nurses themselves, have had a stake in its development and it is the power play between these different bodies that has shaped its identity. As a number of authors have argued, the state is a powerful influence on nursing (Gavin, 1997; MacDonald, 1995). Indeed, by professionalizing certain types of behaviour as in registration, codes of conduct and recommending certain types of intervention, the state has a presence in therapeutic relationships. Moreover, the medical profession and other groups allied to medicine have a bearing on what nurses say, do and think. The nursing profession does not have 'autonomous control over the occupational infrastructure of nursing', and even the content of its educational programmes is substantially influenced by others (Witz, 1992, p. 166).

In relation to the other influences on it, nursing has a 'capillary' structure. By this we mean that it has drawn itself into the gaps left by other disciplines. Nursing also carries on where other disciplines finish; for example, a surgeon finishes the operation but the care of the post-operative patient then commences. In a sense, as a relative newcomer on the scene, nursing has succeeded remarkably well in fitting itself into those spaces where sufferers themselves, their families, their doctors and other care staff cannot reach. As well as being fluid enough to reach the needs that other caring professions cannot deal with, it is also the cement that glues them together. In a patient's 'career' through treatment they might be seen by general practitioners, surgeons, anaesthetists and occupational therapists, but this is all done through a matrix of nursing. Perhaps another indication of this quality is the way that nurses so readily find their way into a whole variety of roles in the health care system. That is, they sometimes turn into managers, executives, lecturers, counsellors, psychotherapists, to name but a few career destinations, and may work in a variety of settings, in hospitals or communities. This diversity of roles for nurses, however, intersects with a range of other professional and political interest groups.

The current vogue for 'evidence-based practice' is problematic. The research that provides the evidence for practice often comes from disciplines outside nursing, such as psychology. For example, family therapy, which is promoted as an effective intervention by psychologists, is now being encouraged for use by nurses, social workers and occupational therapists. The problem is that sometimes we have no evidence that it works when applied by these latter groups of workers. Likewise, even nursing-led interventions that work in the rarefied atmosphere of a prestigious teaching hospital may not be so effective elsewhere. Nurses not only need to be cautious about having their work constructed by ideas from outside groups but also from those formulated within the nursing profession.

There are a great many bodies and interest groups who wish to co-opt and control nursing. As the voiceover in the 1970s film *Close Encounters of the Third Kind* reminded us, 'We are not alone'. Rather like the extraterrestrial aliens in the film, these other presences are not always reassuring. They may be hostile, coercive or invasive. The debate about whether nurses should remain handmaids to doctors is well known, and has been going on for many years. More recently, the cast of language in the health services has become more orientated towards money and management. As we indicated when discussing Traynor's work on management in the health service in chapter 5, nurses increasingly have to justify what they are doing in terms of time and cost-effectiveness.

This relates to an important aspect of what we hope the reader will have learned from this book. Because the work of nursing is primarily linguistic in nature, our intentions have been partly subversive. Nurses must learn to work between the lines of official language to carve out a niche for themselves. This active process is often missed out when scholars attempt to identify what is important to the role of a nurse. All too often it is thought of as merely a matter of interviewing a few nurses to see what they say. This does indeed tell you something useful, but it is altogether too static a model – as if the dynamics of the career could ever be so simply described. Interviews, for example, are unlikely to tell you about the struggles of different professionals to colonize new terrain with their language, definitions and concepts.

There are a variety of ways in which a profession may assert its identity. One strong tendency in the nursing literature we read when preparing the manuscript of this book was to do with the question of professional identity and professional ideology (e.g. Fagermoen, 1997; Taylor, 1997). This quest for an identity, for words and concepts with which to make sense of nursing tends to draw on a relatively static notion of professionalism. That is, it involves an idea of people joining the profession, developing a set of technical skills, acquiring the vocabulary and coming to identify their work as a kind of social role. This is a peculiarly static notion because it does not devote much attention to the way that nurses are continually involved in reconstructing and renegotiating their identities. As we have shown, there is a good deal of evidence of people telling rich and complex stories about how they act as nurses when dealing with patients, doctors and managers, and when being interviewed by researchers. This does not necessarily reflect a monolithic professional identity but is perhaps best seen as reflecting the variety and flexibility that are possible with language. Even if there is a professional identity, a good deal of talk revolves around deciding how to apply it in this particular context. We can see this at work when controversial issues are discussed. For example, is it appropriate to provide electronic tags for elderly patients in case they wander? Should nurses be involved in euthanasia? Or should nurses have the right to opt out of treatments of which they disapprove, like ECT, abortion or compulsory feeding of people with eating disorders? These issues, certainly, are discussed with reference to professional identity and values, yet they are also closely bound up with the treatments themselves. Rather than viewing nurses in terms of a single professional identity, then, it is important to see them as deploying differing identities to make sense of particular issues, controversies or dilemmas. In other words, all this is done through language.

Attempts to develop ideas about professional identity are thus doomed to failure, as this is not readily conceptualized apart from specific activities, conversations or decisions. More general ideals, like the desire to help others, or the desire for work that is challenging and stimulating, are always instantiated by reference to some flesh and blood person whose dressings need changing or who must somehow be prevented from getting bedsores. Nursing, then, is sustained by its details. By contrast, in some literature on the subject of nurses' roles and identities, nurses are rather like cartoon superheroes with their initials emblazoned across their chests, in case other people (or even nurses themselves) do not know who they are or what they are doing. Clearly, everyday life in the clinic or community is not like this. One of the reasons, then, that we have been drawn to language as a means of making sense is that it offers us ways of dealing productively with the chaos and diversity that escape neat professional definitions.

In this book we have deliberately broken out of the typical mould of textbooks. The reader will have noticed by now that we have not developed any neat numbered lists of dos and don'ts. We have certainly drawn attention to the incarcerative potential of language and have expressed concern at the sometimes sloppy way that nursing students use terms like 'clinically depressed'. Yet there is only so much we can do with guidelines and regulations.

Notice that we have stopped short of making specific recommendations as to what the next stage is. Unlike some other bodies, we have not specified guidelines for best practice. Indeed, we have been scathing of attempts to do this. They often concentrate on the trivial – such as the preferred colour of pen – at the expense of the profound consequences that language may have. Moreover, attempts to regulate language use are extremely naïve about the use of language. We have attempted to document the different contexts, themes and styles in language in health care settings and have endeavoured to draw the reader's attention to language in such a way that they can begin to be their own experts on language. The ebb and flow of talk around work settings is constantly changing, forever fascinating and sometimes surprising.

In the face of this, attempts to regulate language tend to address those aspects that are enduring and easy to see. We are left with a set of artefacts like records, computer disks and temperature charts which contain the enduring traces that we can decode. This, however, is only the tip of the iceberg. What is left out is the vast body of language which does the everyday work of nursing. The bulk of this is not technical but mundane. Consequently, it is unlikely that attempts to regulate it can succeed. Such a reductive approach would overlook most of what goes on in nursing.

Efforts to regulate language in any case rely on a misconceived notion of professionalism. It is rare to find the more traditional professions of law, medicine or dentistry relying on detailed protocols for what they are permitted to say, write or respond to. An excess of guidelines immediately marks a profession out as a poor relation, as a body of people who can't be trusted to speak properly.

A further reason why guidelines, lists and protocols are misconceived is that the direction nursing education will take is still uncertain. In the UK nursing has only recently found its place in the academy and begun awarding degrees to nurses. Project 2000 was hailed as a means of strengthening the professional base of nursing, making it more academic and scientific. But nursing assumed all these benefits were coming its way without any costs. The reality is that academic institutions now control entry to the profession, numbers have drastically reduced and disciplines other than nursing are now involved in the teaching of nurses.

Already concerns have emerged that nurses educated under these new training programmes are not all that they were hoped to be. A recent report compiled by researchers at the University of Manchester (1996) on the future of the health care workforce noted that 'there is increasing questioning (not evidence) of the ability of new graduates and Project 2000 diplomates to perform satisfactorily in the clinical environment' (p. 92). This report takes its place among a number of increasingly strong voices demanding a return to a model of training for nurses which is vocational rather than academic, and based not on conceptual understanding but on competencies, rather like the current system of vocational training for other trades in the UK, the NVQ.

Consequently, the direction nurse training will take in the future is uncertain. The different philosophies of what nursing is and how it is done each have their own implications for language use. The future of nursing will depend upon its language and how we use it. In order to explore what this means let us examine two possible directions that language use in nursing may take. As this is the conclusion, the reader will, we hope, forgive us if we are unashamedly partisan.

The two approaches reflect two very different philosophies of nursing, and indeed of language itself. The first is based in a philosophy of standardization and control, the second is based in a reliance on the analytical skills of the nurse as an independent professional.

Scenario 1: Standardization, Regulation and Control

The first, and perhaps the most sinister, of the possible future approaches to language in nursing is the introduction of a standardized language for nursing practice which assumes that the complexity of nursing can be reduced to a set of classifications and definitions and that these can be applied unproblematically. However, the strategy to enforce standardization is beset with contradictions.

To demonstrate what we mean let us examine a current example of this tendency. The International Council of Nurses (ICN) has recently published its 'Alpha Version' of *The International Classification for*

Nursing Practice (ICNP; International Council of Nurses, 1996), in which they claim to provide the beginnings of 'a universal language to define and describe nursing practice' that will form 'the nursing profession's next advance' (p. 1). As the reader might well anticipate, we are highly sceptical about such inflated and naïve claims. What we find particularly distasteful is the overriding vision of control which seems to propel the authors: 'Data collected by using this tool will provide the knowledge necessary for researching, teaching and implementing cost-effective delivery of quality nursing care' (p. 9). Indeed, they promote the adoption of this classificatory system within nurse education: 'Nurse teachers could teach the importance of specifying the nursing diagnoses and nursing interventions within the processes of clinical decision-making and nursing documentation' (p. 223). In other words they see it as desirable to bring the plurality of nursing under a tighter regime of what does and does not count as nursing. They claim that the ICNP 'arose out of concern that nursing's inability to name the patient problems with which nursing was concerned and nursing's distinctive contribution to solving or alleviating them, was preventing nursing from being properly recognised in health care financing' (p. 9). This obviously springs from a deep-seated fear that if nurses do not account for themselves in a way that meets market demands their already limited power base will be further eroded. This fear is justified, of course, because in a market economy, which health care now is, everything has to be costed. Merely stating 'caring for the patient' is not sufficient, because everyone employed in health care does this. For example doctors, physiotherapists and occupational therapists can all claim this rather general function. It is itemizing what is done and how it is described that matters to health care accountants. Thus again we can see how circumstances outside nursing have dictated this move.

While the ICN argue rather convincingly for the necessity of 'some standardization of language' in order for 'concepts to be shared', what they do in fact is smuggle in a pernicious strategy for regulating nursing along far narrower lines. This strategy has more to do with the financial rationalization of nursing via computer-based data collection than consolidating the rich diversity of nursing practices. While the ICN claim that standardization of nursing language 'does not in any way imply the standardisation of nursing practice', such a view is at best naïve and at worst dishonest (p. 24) – clearly the ICN *is* trying to change nursing practice through making prescriptions about its language.

Despite the usefulness of *some* kinds of definition, many of those proposed in the ICNP border on the ridiculous, and rather than increasing nursing's scientific profile tend to trivialize it. For example, 'moving' is defined in the following terms: 'Self Care: Moving is a Nursing Phenomena pertaining to Activity of Daily Living with the following specific characteristics: Effective basic action of moving oneself' (p. 53). Or, even more ludicrous: 'Water is a Nursing Phenomena pertaining to the Physical Environment with the following specific characteristics: [we can barely control our suspense!] A colourless transparent odourless, tasteless liquid compound of oxygen and hydrogen found in seas, lakes, rivers and underground necessary for the survival of individuals' (p. 58). Even worse, the document lists the most mundane objects that nurses use or work with, for example, soap, knives, forks, spoons and televisions! The ICN suggest that nurses might use the ICNP as a kind of 'telephone directory' which the practising nurse can use to better describe what they do. It is beginning to look more like a mail-order catalogue.

The ICNP stresses the usefulness of international agreement or standardization of nursing language as if this is possible or practicable. The ICNP 'cross-maps' its own definitions with a selection of others. For example, we find 'cross-mappings' of terms such as NANDA's 'Impaired gas exchange' with ICNP's alternative 'Ineffective Gas Exchange' (p. 158). The question is: where do you stop once this kind of labyrinthine activity is initiated? There can be no end to the variations in terminologies or interpretations of them.

A further reason why we are dissatisfied about this approach to regulating nursing language is that it does not address many of the concerns we have raised in this book. Simply standardizing language does not reduce its incarcerative potential. As we have seen, there are a range of features of language in the clinic which actively construct identities for patients, as 'prostitutes', as 'violent' or as elderly persons meriting secondary baby talk. Delimiting the legitimate terms does not remedy this situation.

These attempts to standardize the terminology and language of nursing are aligned with the ambition on the part of some of those involved in the discipline to see it reformulated as a set of technical skills or competencies and make it once again a vocational rather than an academic discipline.

There is, of course, a continuum between two excesses – on the one hand idiosyncratic non-standardization and, on the other, totalitarian standardization. We believe that both extremes are unacceptable. In this book we have been concerned to show the dangers of unethical language use in nursing and have placed great emphasis on the needs for individual practitioners to adopt a sophisticated approach to the language they employ. This is hand in glove with the value of reflective practice. Only by carefully monitoring their individual language actions are nurses able to become reflective practitioners.

This interest in reflective practice which has been growing in nursing for the past 15 years or so leads on to another, more optimistic vision of the future, in relation to the concerns we have raised. By reflective language practice, incarcerative and other inappropriate language can be minimized. These issues have been conspicuously absent from the kind of focus that the ICN adopts. For all the rhetoric of inclusion, for example by mentioning international consultation practices, the ICNP is embedded within a Euro-American world view. The move to standardization ignores several important issues – for example, the way that language is a constructive rather than a descriptive medium; the whole issue of the power nurses wield through language – and it ignores how nurses are being subjected to external powers, edicts and constraints.

We hope to have shown the limitations of an approach to language in clinical practice which attempts to define, limit and regulate what can be said or written. Let us now elaborate on a second scenario for the future which takes full advantage of the critical skills of the nurse.

SCENARIO 2: REFLECTIVE PRACTICE – DEEPENING LANGUAGE AWARENESS, ENHANCING UNDERSTANDING

Language enables us to describe and potentially to transform aspects of our work. One of the hallmarks of any profession is that its members engage in debate with each other about aspects of their work. Progress and growth are the positive outcomes of reflective practices, embodied in increased choices and increased professional awareness. For nursing to achieve these ends, it must regularly and vigorously examine its practices and the values that underpin them, and the public's expectations of nurses and nursing care. Where there is no examination of practice and underlying theory, a profession stagnates – 'if you always do what you have always done, you will always get what you have always got'. The past few years have seen increasing reflection on what it means to be a nurse and what the effects of nursing activity are. The considerable increase in recent years in the number of conferences, seminars and journals for nurses bears witness to the urgency of critical inquiry that is currently taking place within nursing.

The roots of recent reflective practice can be found in the works of such writers as Freire (1972) and Illich (1977) (Jarvis, 1992). The ideas of these writers arose out of their experience as individuals working with very impoverished peoples in Third World countries who felt powerless and trapped. Their aim was to show people that by themselves they may feel powerless, but as communities and movements they could be very effective. Their work was later to be referred to as Liberation Theology or the Politics of Resistance. The ideas contained in these works were brought together in a book entitled *The Reflective Practitioner* written by Schon (1983). Its contents were taken very seriously by professions who had difficulty reconciling theory and practice. The goal of reflective practice, argued Schon, was to change indeterminate situations into determinate ones. This is akin to consciousness raising in that it involves the development of concepts, languages and means of talking about what was previously hidden or tacit. Fundamental to all this is a belief that people can actually effect change. Such ideology is ineffective if people do not believe they have the power to do this.

The fruitfulness of this increasing reflection on practice is essentially dependent on the degree to which nurses can increase their awareness of the language they use to describe their work and professional aspirations, and their understanding of the lineage of the terms and expressions that have become the accepted currency of nursing debate. The language of nursing contains a good many terms imported from other disciplines such as medicine, psychology and management. During the 1990s particularly, the language of nursing was infused with changes resulting from a market-driven health service, users' movements and professional expansionism. The current focus on reflective practice attempts to address the problem of definition within nursing. In other words, a major problem in trying to define the unique enterprise of nursing is that the language available to describe it is often derived from disciplines outside nursing. Reflective practice inclines nurses to examine these alien influences that consolidate the external control of nursing practice. It also assists nurses in uncovering and challenging their own personal values and prejudices.

If we are to take the challenge of reflective practice seriously, this will involve addressing nursing on a number of fronts. Nurses need to become increasingly aware of the textually transmitted values currently being communicated in nursing. Nurses need to examine more critically the language that is used to describe their practice rather than passively accepting regulated vocabularies and categories about what it is they do. Reflective practice, at its best, can enable us to understand the controlling influence of language. Moreover, it can empower nurses to resist contemporary threats to the core values of nursing which come via language couched in management terms, and resist threats to the profession posed by naive schemes to try to define all the words in nurses' vocabularies. Without this reflective ability nursing may become the instrument of politically driven health agendas which promote a task-focused service, which does not sit very well with the caring, compassionate philosophy nursing has always prided itself on.

The importance of being aware of and sensitive to the language used to describe nursing work and the heavy burden of meanings which it carries has been emphasized in previous chapters. Nurses have made considerable strides since the 1950s and 1960s, when they began to identify unique aspects of their role, to the 1970s and 1980s, when they defined and asserted the skills base of their profession, to the early 1990s, when they started to explore and try to understand the diverse and increasingly complex legal, ethical and professional issues surrounding their work. The willingness and ability to analyse nursing conceptually from different perspectives require a high degree of competence in the use of technical languages and familiarity with the meanings they convey.

To examine the theoretical and practice bases of contemporary nursing is an intellectual task of considerable magnitude which has only recently become of interest and importance to nurses, both those working in academic life and those in the clinical arena. An eagerness to reflect on aspects of one's work, to engage in debate about its theory and practice is a sign of maturity in a profession that has a sense of the value of its contribution to health care. Traditionally, a positivist epistemology assisted nurses in acquiring knowledge of their work, a kind of knowledge that Schon (1983) has referred to as the 'high hard ground' of the profession's understanding of itself. This appears to be the philosophy that propels the attempts to define nursing terms, equipment and diagnoses which we criticized above. In a similar spirit, Brykczynska (1995) criticizes the naïvety of this philosophy for assuming that the learning that takes place in the classroom or the lecture theatre can be transferred into the clinical setting and will there prove to be relevant to the problems that nurses face. In reality, the everyday practice of nursing is more a question of 'the swampy lowlands' (Schon, 1983) rather than the high, hard ground. Nurses encounter complex and distressing problems which defy solutions based on classroom knowledge or preformulated lists of categories.

Brykczynska (1995) argues that reflective practice is a means of thinking about oneself in the world, about the impact that the world has on the practitioner and about the impact that the practitioner has on the world. To be able to be truly reflective practitioners, she argues, nurses need to make a huge leap forward in the way they think about and act in their professional roles. Reflective practice requires nurses to become sceptics in a way that would have been entirely foreign and incomprehensible to their ancestors of even a few decades ago; they are required to be sceptical about the way in which they deliver care, the knowledge that underpins it, the power relationships that drive it. They are required to ask sceptical questions such as: 'What do I know?', 'How do I know it?', 'Is it the best knowledge available?', 'Have I evidence of my own to confirm or refute it?' The reflective approach demands that every aspect of the individual's nursing practice should be subjected to critical scrutiny in order to justify the care being provided. It is through such rigorous inquiry that nurses increase their awareness of and insight into the values, beliefs and motives of patients, clients and carers and are ultimately able to offer a service that is tailored to the unique needs of individuals rather than to the presumed needs of groups.

The importance of having a critical mass of nurses – and this mass must include the vast majority of practitioners – who are able to reflect on what they are doing and to articulate the essence of nursing cannot be underestimated. The nursing core needs to be exposed, defined and defended if it is to withstand the attacks on care currently being mounted by market forces within health care. It is by becoming more aware of the ideas being absorbed into nursing and the language used to describe them that nurses become more secure within their profession and more able to take issue with and resist ideologies that threaten the integrity of their profession. Nurses should be able, as a result of their education and their critical engagement in practice, to assert the primacy of nursing in the health care arena and the major contribution it makes to treatment, cure and health promotion. There may be a considerable number of nurses, particularly those employed in the hospital sector, who are lacking in confidence to assert the centrality of nursing care and insecure about what it is they are defending. This may be due to the dominance of medical values in the hospital setting and to the way in which nurses, almost inevitably, internalize those values when they work in hospitals. Reflective practice may assist these nurses in rediscovering their obligations *as nurses* rather than as assistants to doctors and in recognizing that where nursing becomes subordinate to other forms of care the client is receiving an inferior service.

GROUNDING REFLECTIVE PRACTICE: FROM PHILOSOPHY TO POLITICS

Given our intention to examine some aspects of the future of language in nursing, the reader may be surprised by what follows. We will begin this section with an excursion into the past. However, it is important that we become aware of this particular philosophical past as it undergirds the current vogue for reflection in nursing today. In order for the reflective practice of contemporary nurses to reach its full potential we should explore how it originated. Present-day reflective heresies can trace their genealogy back to the paradigm-shifting controversies of the Middle Ages. Few nurses nowadays would take issue with the currently accepted belief that nursing practice is based on humanistic values which respect persons and promote human dignity (Brykczynska, 1995). In the popular imagination, nursing is associated with caring; that it is person centred, altruistic and empowering. Nurses eagerly identify with such notions and tend to explain their work in terms of what they assume humanistic care to be. And yet it has not always been so self evident. As Brykczynska (1995) observes, few nurses have a proper understanding of what humanism is about, its origins, the ideas of the philosophers associated with it and the history of its influence on and adoption into nursing and nursing language.

The history of humanism and humanistic thinking is a long one and, as a philosophy, it has been used at different times to justify political regimes, actions and care management that have been far from beneficial to human beings. Humanistic approaches are often associated with the Kantian ethic that people should never be used as a means to an end but always treated as an end in themselves. The attractiveness of this moral high ground has exerted a powerful influence on those engaged in 'people services'. However, all too often caring professionals have acted on the arguably distorted humanistic premise that the care offered to people will be in their best interests if professionals believe it to be so. Reflective practice aims to take health carers beyond the humanistic rhetoric of mission statements, care plans and fashionable therapies to far deeper levels of understanding where multiple interpretations of how care is defined, specified, delivered, received and interpreted are possible.

Brykczynska (1995) attempts to lay bare the complexities of the term 'humanism' through an exploration of its manifestations in history, literature, religion and philosophy. Intellectual revolutions, she contends, have always been driven by people who possessed the ability to analyse the context of their own times in the light of history and with a vision of how they would like the future to be shaped. Duns Scotus, Thomas Aquinas, William Occam and Thomas More were intellectual revolutionaries who possessed the complementary skills of being able to reflect on society and then to express their reflections through the spoken or written word. These 'change agents' were equally well educated in the arts and the sciences, but were not hidebound by the accepted ways of thinking and behaving of their era.

The width of scholarship presented by Brykczynska (1995) concludes with an examination of how recent philosophers, such as Sartre, Husserl, Heidegger, Kierkegaard and others have extended our understanding of the term 'humanism' and in so doing influenced much of current nursing theory and practice. The incorporation, by some educational institutions, of the arts and humanities into nursing curricula draw heavily on those authors who inquire into such areas as, 'What is it to be human'?, 'To what extent can humans shape themselves and their future'?, 'What is it to live a fulfilled life?', 'How best can one cope with a sense of aloneness'? and 'How do humans view their own frailty and death'? Perhaps the philosopher with the greatest influence on nursing recently has been Sartre, who espouses the position that 'man is nothing else but his own plan; and he exists only to the extent that he fulfils himself. He is nothing more or less than his own life. (1989, p. 25)' People must create for themselves their own authentic being; they must realize their potential and resist all attempts to subject themselves to the will of others, however well intentioned.

Reflective practice is much more than merely thinking about one's work. It is made possible precisely because of this intellectual history. What we take for granted about the nature of care and the value of human happiness has been struggled over in the past. The present-day construct of reflective practice assumes that there are systems of thought which underpin practice and that those engaged in practical nursing benefit from revisiting these from time to time.

Reflective practice seeks to identify problems, inconsistencies, and areas where there is no theoretical base, in order to assist individuals to cope with the work they are being asked to do. The original humanistic formulation of reflective practice is that individuals are helped to achieve personal growth in their work. This view of reflection can be profitably opened up further by attention to the issues we have addressed in this book. Until now, reflective practice has not had the precise intellectual tools to do the job it was charged with. What we hope to have left the reader with is a sense that the rich seam of language at work can be mined in order to fathom out what it is that nursing and other health care disciplines are achieving.

A key characteristic of nursing is its openness to diversity and its ability to deploy diverse tactics in an attempt to promote patient well-being within the political confines of its own professional and institutional status. To classify nursing narrowly is to miss what is paradigmatic of nursing: its non-resolution, its non-totalization, its defiance of end- gaining. It is not the capacity to cure *per se* which is valuable to nursing practice but the ability of nurses to shift their social performance from moment to moment in a perceived helping of others. The success or failure of nursing practices can only ever be partially demonstrated. Ultimately, therefore, in the great majority of cases the success or failure of nursing remains imponderable, unexcavated or unexcavatable. The accountability of nursing will always remain incomplete. What needs to be accounted for, then, is its ability to be diverse in its responses. It is the nature of nursing to be forever incomplete or non-totalizable. What should be valued in nursing is its defiance of set, rigid, and totalitarian trends. If nursing succumbs to the values of the marketplace, it will abdicate its unique contribution to health care. It must resist the inquisition of the marketplace and not slavishly give into it. By promoting its heretical difference, nursing may succeed in challenging the prevailing market orthodoxies and moderating their deficiencies.

It may be that nurses find the idea of taking a stand on language issues rather daunting. This is to be expected. After all, there is a lot at stake and there are some powerful players formulating the language and hence the practice of nursing. We hope that individual nurses can take away with them two broad principles to guide their future language activity. Firstly, by reflecting on how they produce texts and receive the texts of others, they may be better placed to intervene in the way nursing care is constructed and implemented. Secondly, a more sophisticated and politicized understanding of the social operations of language can only benefit the nursing profession in determining the importance of its unique contribution among other competing health care approaches. This may involve the development of a more confident and distinctive language 'which opposes the impersonal, spiritually divested and mechanistic arena of the "free" yet highly "oppressive" marketplace.' Nurses 'need to assess the balance between their responsibilities as employees and their spiritual responsibilities to clients' (Nolan and Crawford, 1997, p. 293). We hope that as a result of reading this book nurses will be encouraged to be 'incurably informed' about language issues and will refuse to say, write, listen or read without reflecting critically on the social consequences of these activities in communicating care.

REFERENCES

Brykczynska, G. (1995) Humanism: a weak link in nursing theory, in *Towards Advanced Nursing Practice* (eds J.E.Schober and J.M. Hinchliff), Arnold, London.

Fagermoen, M.S. (1997) Professional identity: values embedded in meaningful nursing practice. *Journal of Advanced Nursing*, 25, 434–41.

Freire, P. (1972) *Pedagogy of the Oppressed*, Penguin, Harmondsworth.

Gavin, J.N. (1997) Nursing ideology and the 'generic carer'. *Journal of Advanced Nursing*, 26, 692–7.

Illich, I. (1977) *Disabling Professions*, Marian Boyars, London.

Conclusion

International Council of Nurses (1996) *The International Classification for Nursing Practice*, Alpha Version, International Council of Nurses, Geneva.

Jarvis, P. (1992) Reflective practice. *Nurse Education Today*, **12**, 174–81.

MacDonald, K.M. (1995) *The Sociology of the Professions*, Sage, London.

Nolan, P. and Crawford, P. (1997) Towards a rhetoric of spirituality in mental health care. *Journal of Advanced Nursing*, **26**, 289–94.

Sartre, J.P. (1989) *Existentialism and Humanism*, Methuen, London.

Schon, T. (1983) *The Reflective Practitioner*, Basic Books, New York.

Taylor, J.S. (1997) Nursing ideology: identification and legitimation. *Journal of Advanced Nursing*, **25**, 442–6.

University of Manchester (1996) *The Future Health-Care Workforce*, University of Manchester, Manchester.

Witz, A. (1992) *Professions and Patriarchy*, Routledge, London.

INDEX

Index

Index